KIDNEY DISEASE

KIDNEY
—DISEASE—

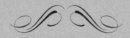

A Guide *for* Living

WALTER A. HUNT

Foreword by
Ronald D. Perrone, M.D.
Tufts Medical Center

THE JOHNS HOPKINS UNIVERSITY PRESS
Baltimore

NOTES TO THE READER. This book is not meant to substitute for medical care of people with kidney disease, and treatment should not be based solely on its contents. Instead, treatment must be developed in a dialogue between the individual and his or her physician. Our book has been written to help with that dialogue.

The author and publisher have made reasonable efforts to determine that the selection and dosage of drugs discussed in this text conform to the practices of the general medical community. The medications described do not necessarily have specific approval by the U.S. Food and Drug Administration for use in the diseases and dosages for which they are recommended. In view of ongoing research, changes in governmental regulations, and the constant flow of information relating to drug therapy and drug reactions, the reader is urged to check the package insert of each drug for any change in indications and dosage and for warnings and precautions. This is particularly important when the recommended agent is a new and/or infrequently used drug.

© 2011 The Johns Hopkins University Press
All rights reserved. Published 2011
Printed in the United States of America on acid-free paper
2 4 6 8 9 7 5 3 1

The Johns Hopkins University Press
2715 North Charles Street
Baltimore, Maryland 21218-4363
www.press.jhu.edu

Library of Congress Cataloging-in-Publication Data
Hunt, W. A. (Walter A.)
Kidney disease : a guide for living / Walter A. Hunt ; foreword by Ronald D. Perrone.
p. cm.
Includes bibliographical references and index.
ISBN-13: 978-0-8018-9963-8 (hardcover : alk. paper)
ISBN-10: 0-8018-9963-X (hardcover : alk. paper)
ISBN-13: 978-0-8018-9964-5 (pbk. : alk. paper)
ISBN-10: 0-8018-9964-8 (pbk. : alk. paper)
1. Kidneys—Diseases—Popular works. 2. Kidneys—Diseases—Treatment—Popular works. I. Title.
RC902.H85 2011
616.6′1—dc22   2010025286

A catalog record for this book is available from the British Library.

Figures 2.1, 3.3, 3.4, 3.5, 6.3, 6.4, 6.5, 6.6, 6.7, 6.8, 6.9, 6.10, 6.11, 6.12, 6.13, 6.14, 7.4, and 7.5 are by Jacqueline Schaffer.

Special discounts are available for bulk purchases of this book. For more information, please contact Special Sales at 410-516-6936 or specialsales@press.jhu.edu.

The Johns Hopkins University Press uses environmentally friendly book materials, including recycled text paper that is composed of at least 30 percent post-consumer waste, whenever possible. All of our book papers are acid-free, and our jackets and covers are printed on paper with recycled content.

CONTENTS

Foreword, by Ronald D. Perrone, M.D.   *vii*
Preface   *xi*

Chapter 1
UNDERSTANDING KIDNEY FAILURE   1

Chapter 2
WHAT KIDNEYS DO   16

Chapter 3
WHY KIDNEYS FAIL   24

Chapter 4
DIAGNOSING AND MANAGING
KIDNEY DISEASE   49

Chapter 5
PREVENTING AND POSTPONING
KIDNEY FAILURE   65

Chapter 6

DIALYSIS   80

Chapter 7

TRANSPLANTATION   118

Chapter 8

FUTURE TREATMENT OPTIONS   149

EPILOGUE   159

Notes   *161*
Glossary   *163*
Resources   *171*
Index   *179*

FOREWORD

It is a pleasure to write this foreword. Very few books like this one are available for people diagnosed with kidney disease. Medical information about kidney disease and kidney failure is abundant, yet important perspectives from patients who have actually experienced kidney disease, kidney failure, and resulting dialysis and transplantation are not easily obtained. Walter Hunt has provided careful and understandable explanations for the layperson, and he's offered his personal experience with and perspectives on how kidney failure has affected his life. I congratulate him for providing this excellent guide for people with kidney disease.

I made the decision to enter the field of nephrology during my second year of medical school while doing a rotation on the inpatient nephrology service. Witnessing the miracle of transplantation and the life-saving treatment of dialysis encouraged me because I recognized that, as a physician, I would have these tools to help patients overcome serious illness. Before these treatments became available, kidney failure was a disease with very limited therapeutic options.

Working with people newly diagnosed with kidney disease and with people who have been living with kidney disease for a long time provides tremendous opportunities to influence their care.

When I meet newly diagnosed people, my hope for them is, first, to provide a specific and accurate diagnosis. Then, if a treatment is available, I implement treatment to slow the progress of the disease. It is important to educate patients at this stage, to inform them and their families about the disease, and to enlist the family's participation in the patient's care. If necessary, I begin treatment to prevent and manage potential complications and provide reassurance about the options for therapy, including dialysis and transplantation. All of this is not easily accomplished during a single visit! The relationship between patient and doctor is a long-term one with multiple opportunities for my patients to ask questions and to receive information from print or electronic sources to help them understand and manage their disease.

Follow-up visits provide patients and me additional opportunities to go over their care, to discuss how they are doing for their part of the care, and to solidify the bond of comfort and trust that occurs with a long-term doctor-patient relationship. At these visits I often have another opportunity to interact with additional family members as well. Different stages of the disease require different interventions. Long periods of stability are gratifying for everyone involved and don't necessarily require long discussions or any intervention; in contrast, the approach of end-stage renal failure and the need for dialysis or transplant can provoke much anxiety and require frequent visits for education, counseling, and medication adjustment.

Receiving a diagnosis of kidney disease is frightening for nearly everyone. Vivid fears of dialysis and rapid progression to kidney failure are common. More often than not, there are interventions to slow the progression of chronic kidney disease and to manage the complications. Although these interventions are not cures—in the way that an antibiotic can cure pneumonia—they can be helpful in preserving health.

I believe it is important for individuals with kidney disease to be fully engaged in the management of their disease. When patients are engaged and involved, it's more likely that the progression of the disease will be slowed and complications will be prevented. There are multiple opportunities for patients to improve their long-term outcome. They can become educated about the disease, take appropriate medication and manage their diet, obtain a home blood pressure device and regularly measure and report blood pressure, join patient support groups, and support research and educational efforts by foundations like the National Kidney Foundation and the Polycystic Kidney Disease Foundation.

Dialysis is not a perfect treatment for kidney failure, but, nonetheless, it is life saving and can provide a reasonable quality of life for individuals. Improvements in dialysis technology and the increasing availability of home dialysis and daily dialysis treatments have led to much better outcomes for many individuals. Transplantation, while not a cure for kidney disease, is an excellent treatment, yet it still requires frequent visits to medical providers, lots of pills, and potentially serious complications from these potent medications. Greatly improved quality of life and longer life result from this intervention, but careful compliance and follow-up are necessary.

As a physician who has not personally experienced kidney disease, my understanding of the terrifying nature of receiving a diagnosis of kidney disease has always come to me secondhand. In *Kidney Disease: A Guide for Living,* Walter Hunt provides an honest perspective of someone who has experienced loss of kidney function, had years of dialysis, and received a successful transplant. These insights and personal experiences, along with explanations of biology and medical treatment, are a tremendous resource. The reassurance provided by someone "who has been there" will, I hope, decrease the anxiety for those who are newly diagnosed or are facing new treatments like dialysis or transplantation.

It is my hope that you will use this book for guidance and companionship as you journey through the complexities of the diagnosis and treatment of chronic kidney disease.

Ronald D. Perrone, M.D.
Associate Chief, Division of Nephrology
Tufts Medical Center

PREFACE

Nearly 550,000 people in the United States suffer from chronic kidney failure and require dialysis or transplantation to live. I am one of them. I inherited a genetic defect that caused cysts to form in my kidneys, eventually destroying my kidney function. For ten years I dealt with kidney failure, including more than seven years on dialysis and numerous complications, before receiving a successful kidney transplant. Called polycystic kidney disease (PKD), the genetic defect I have is the fourth leading cause of kidney failure in the United States. People with PKD have a 50 percent chance of inheriting it from an affected parent. My mother and sister had PKD and ultimately died from complications of the disease.

When I first realized that my kidneys might fail, I searched for resources that would help me prepare for what was to come. Plenty of information was available describing kidney disease and the ways doctors treat kidney failure. However, I could not find a systematic discussion of what it would be like to experience kidney failure and its treatment. My doctors were not able to help me imagine what the experience would be like. Although a doctor can be empathetic when interacting with patients, unless he has personally experienced kidney failure, a doctor's perspective of kidney failure is largely a medical one, not a personal one.

I decided to write this book to provide a service for other people like me, people wanting practical information about what causes kidney failure, how patients can help themselves cope both physically and emotionally, and what factors can help them make personal health care decisions. Information helps people make better decisions, potentially leading to better outcomes, and helps them feel more in control of their condition—both of which provide a better quality of life. Although I am not a physician, my thirty-year career in medical research helps me understand the science behind kidney failure and the treatments available. Also, over the years I have learned how to cope with many of the problems of kidney failure. It is my sincere hope that this book will assist you in coming to terms with your own unique situation.

After first covering the basics of how kidneys function (chapters 1 and 2), why kidneys can fail (chapter 3), the diagnosis and management of kidney failure (chapter 4), and strategies to reduce kidney deterioration (chapter 5), I discuss the two treatment options for kidney failure: dialysis (chapter 6) and transplantation (chapter 7). In chapter 8, I describe promising treatments that are being developed and that one day may change the course of kidney disease. Throughout the book I include citations to other publications that you may wish to consult for further discussion of specific topics. A list of resources appears at the end of the book. Because the meaning of some of the scientific terms may be difficult to remember from chapter to chapter, a glossary is included that defines key words.

Throughout the book I discuss my personal treatment decisions. When considering dialysis, did I want to control my treatment on my own schedule at home, or have someone else do it for me at a dialysis center, on their schedule? In the case of transplantation, was I willing to compromise my immune system for the rest of my life and risk developing infections and even cancer in exchange for a better quality of life? Ultimately, I had to decide for myself. You will, too. I discuss the pros and cons of each treatment, based on my own experience and scientific research, to help you decide, with your doctor, what is best for you.

When I present scientific information related to kidney disease, I have tried to write in a way that makes this information understandable to everyone, including people with no scientific training. It's worth repeating that educating yourself about your disease can make a big difference in preparing yourself for your future treatment. Realizing that you have the right and the ability to choose will be a major asset in having a say in your medical treatment. If you are grounded in sufficient knowledge to know what questions to ask, you will be in a better position to contribute to your treatment. Having choices, even when they are not always good ones, is empowering. This book will put you in a better position to make more informed choices.

I could not have completed this book without the support and advice of the many people who read drafts of the manuscript, including Dr. Bob Craig, Bobbie Festa, Nancy Hayes, Linda Howerton, Julia Roberts, Dr. Bernie Rabin, and Howard Jung, Jr. In addition, I would like to thank Jill McMaster and Dr. Y. Nabil Yakub for reviewing early versions of the book.

Special thanks are owed to Dr. Ronald Perrone. Ron shared many hours of his time explaining kidney failure from a doctor's perspective and making sure that the information in this book is accurate. He did so with good cheer and clear explanations. Any inaccuracies that may have crept in after his thorough reviews are my sole responsibility. I greatly appreciate Ron's time, scholarship, and collegial spirit in bringing this book to fruition.

Finally, I wish to thank the Johns Hopkins University Press for supporting this project, especially my editor, Jacqueline Wehmueller. Her skill, support, and advice were indispensable in creating the final work. It was great working with her.

KIDNEY DISEASE

I

UNDERSTANDING KIDNEY FAILURE

On August 11, 1997, a catheter was implanted in my abdomen so I could receive dialysis. My kidneys had failed. I could still urinate, but I couldn't eliminate all the waste products that I accumulated from food. It's natural to take urinating for granted—it's something we've done since the day we were born! As adults we think about going to the bathroom only when we can't get to one because we're trapped in a business meeting, say, or stuck in traffic. And we do not usually discuss urination in polite company. When we need to urinate, we just excuse ourselves or adopt a euphemism—we're going to the powder room or we're going to see a man about a horse.

When urinating is no longer a normal, almost trivial, activity, our lives are altered. When urinating becomes a focus of our attention, our lives are radically changed. When my kidneys started to shut down, I found the prospect of kidney failure overwhelming.

I had so many questions: "Why are my kidneys failing? Is there anything I can do to save my kidneys? How will I know when my kidneys have failed? What will it feel like when my kidneys fail? Is there a cure or treatment for kidney failure?"

The good news, as I found out, is that kidney failure is no longer a death sentence, as it once was. Those of us with kidney failure can still have productive lives. The bad news is that we may spend countless hours going to dialysis and doctors' offices and making sure we take all our medications. There are some aspects of the disease that we can't control. One aspect of the disease that we *can* control is how well we understand it. Understanding kidney failure—what causes it, how it may affect our lives, and what options we have—can help us take an active role in treating our disease, lift our spirits, achieve a better outcome, and improve our quality of life.

How Many People Have It?

The number of people with chronic kidney failure in the United States is rising at an alarming rate. Many of the people being newly diagnosed are developing kidney failure as a consequence of uncontrolled diabetes. The 2010 Annual Data Report issued by the National Institutes of Health indicates that by the end of 2008, nearly 550,000 people in the United States were being treated for chronic kidney failure or end-stage renal disease (ESRD).[1] That same year, doctors diagnosed more than 112,000 new cases of chronic kidney failure.

The primary causes of kidney failure are diabetes, hypertension, glomerular diseases, and polycystic kidney disease (PKD). In table 1.1, you can see the number of people afflicted with these four diseases who also have kidney failure. Figure 1.1 shows the percentage of all people with kidney failure that can be attributed to each

Table 1.1
Kidney Failure in the United States, 2008

Cause	Number of Cases
Diabetes	197,037
Hypertension	127,935
Glomerular diseases	81,599
Polycystic kidneys	24,828
All other causes	87,701
Total	519,100

cause (called *prevalence*) during the same period. Figure 1.2 illustrates how the picture is changing, with more new cases being attributed to diabetes.

Diabetes and hypertension account for 62 percent of the cases of kidney failure. The rest of the cases result from glomerular diseases, polycystic kidney disease, and other causes not reflected in figure 1.1. Alarmingly, the new cases attributed to diabetes and hypertension jumped to 72 percent during 2008 (figure 1.2). Diabetes,

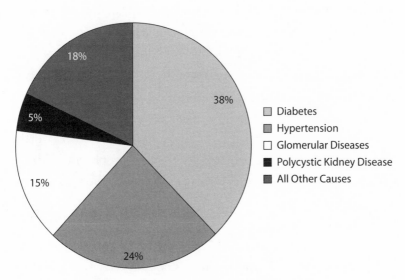

Figure 1.1. Causes of Kidney Failure, 2008

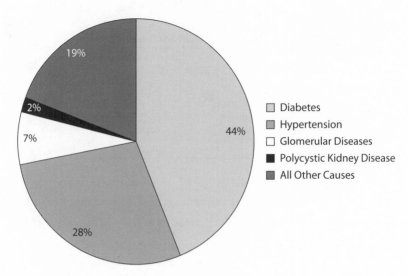

Figure 1.2. New Cases of Kidney Failure, by Cause of Kidney Failure, 2008

the most common cause of kidney failure, accounts for 44 percent of new cases of kidney failure. Because obesity can lead to diabetes and because an increasing number of people are obese or morbidly obese, more people are at risk of kidney failure. The *incidence* of new cases of kidney disease due to diabetes is almost 50,000 each year (slightly lower than in 2007). On the other hand, new cases of glomerular diseases declined to less than 7,500.

In an era when health care costs are being scrutinized, it's worth mentioning that in 2007 the cost of treating people with kidney failure in the United States was more than $26.8 billion per year in Medicare spending.

Disease and Emotions

Discovering that we have a chronic, potentially fatal disease can be overwhelming. It seems that life as we know it has changed, perhaps forever. Sometimes this is true, when we have a disease that doctors can only manage, not treat or cure. Although people with kidney failure require some form of intervention for their entire lives, doctors can manage *and* treat kidney failure.

When I discovered that I had a serious chronic disease, I experienced emotional reactions similar to the six stages of grief related to death as described by Elisabeth Kübler-Ross: fear, denial, anger, bargaining, depression, and, finally, acceptance.[2] Loss of kidney function parallels some aspects of death. Kidney failure can represent the loss of life as we know it. Our reactions might be just as compelling as those of people approaching death, since we are not sure if we will survive. My emotional reactions did not necessarily represent a continuum of responses. They came and went over the course of my disease. Even when I finally accepted my disease, I occasionally became angry and depressed about my condition. At times, I was just tired. However, if I wanted to live, which I did, I *had* to come to terms with all the aspects of kidney failure.

Nearly everyone who has a chronic disease experiences fear and denial. Not knowing what to do can be terrifying and paralyzing. We may know little about our condition and may be afraid of suffering or even dying. Sometimes we may not want to believe that we have a serious illness. People who have spent active lives find it difficult to accept the restrictions placed on many activities that are part of life. It is easier to ignore the problem in hopes that the diagnosis is wrong or that the illness will just go away.

Yet denial serves a useful purpose by rationing only the amount of information and emotion we can process at any given time. Profound loss is difficult for even the strongest people. Denial gives us time to absorb the news of our illness in a measured way. We cannot believe that our kidneys are failing. We feel fine. Later, the significance of what is happening to us becomes more of a reality.

Once we can no longer deny the fact that we have a chronic illness and the full weight of its reality sinks in, we often become angry. Why me? What did I do to deserve this? Could I have done something to prevent my illness? The questions are endless. You might conclude you have been targeted for illness, possibly as some form of punishment. This is not true. Although contracting an illness is not exactly random—many illnesses are influenced by genetic and lifestyle factors—it is not personal, either. We can imagine all kinds of "what if" scenarios. If only we had done something differently, maybe the outcome would have been different. Processing anger can be an important part of emotional healing. Feeling your anger can help you move on.

People who believe in God may try bargaining for a better outcome. If you promise to dedicate the remainder of your life to God's purpose, maybe God will give back your kidney function. In the end, however, it does not matter. The loss is permanent. We have to face the reality of our kidney failure.

When the reality of losing kidney function finally sets in, the emotional responses can deepen, possibly leading to depression, either steady or intermittent. Minor depression—feeling sad—is normal if it does not become too severe. Like denial, depression can allow the brain time to absorb the full impact of the diagnosis. Eventually, after depression has served its purpose, it can dissipate. But more severe depression can make your treatment more difficult, robbing you of the motivation and energy you need to get treatment and take care of yourself. Depression that does not subside is a very serious condition that may require medical attention.

Once you have moved through the stages of fear, denial, anger, bargaining, and depression, you may begin to accept your diagnosis. In time, you will realize that you can no longer avoid kidney disease. It is at this point that you have the greatest opportunity to take control of your health, even if it means your life will never be the same again.

Educating Yourself—and Other Tools for Dealing with Kidney Failure

Not everyone gets a warning that their kidneys are in danger of failing. Some people discover that they have had high blood pressure for a long time without knowing it. For other people, kidneys fail because of diabetes or other causes that could possibly have been prevented.

In my own case, I lived for twenty years knowing my kidneys might fail, but I seldom thought about it seriously. Because my mother and sister had died of complications of PKD I knew I might have the disease, but I did not experience symptoms, other than high blood pressure, until I was almost 45 years old. That was the first time I had to confront my own mortality, and it terrified me. Eventually, I had to accept my fate whether I wanted to or not. Acceptance is something that nearly everyone with kidney disease can achieve.

Like people with other chronic diseases, people with kidney disease must manage their disease every day for the rest of their lives. There are no days off, and no vacations. If we do not treat our failing kidneys, we can become sicker and possibly die. However, once we learn what to do and integrate those lessons into our lives, our lives can become more normal. Life will not be the same as when we were well, but we can still pursue a happy one. It may not seem that way at this point, but during the course of this book, I hope to convince you that your life is not over with kidney failure, and that other opportunities are possible. I will show you how.

First, learn everything you can about your disease. You may not have a medical background, but you should be able to grasp the basics of your disease when they are described in language you understand. This book will introduce you to information that will allow you to have more control over your condition. I found that the more I understood about kidney failure, the less afraid I felt.

There are many sources of information about kidney disease. Start with your doctor. Several kidney disease organizations provide information in accessible language. For more technical information, access the medical literature through the Library of Medicine at the National Institutes of Health in Bethesda, Maryland. (Additional details about such organizations and ways to access the medical literature are provided in the Resources section at the end of this book.)

As I learned more about my disease, I found that I had far less to be concerned about than I thought. There would be tough times, but I knew that with the knowledge that I acquired and with the right attitude, I could make the process of treatment much easier. As a trained scientist, I was able to examine the scientific literature to learn about my disease and I was able to understand what was happening to me. But many scholarly articles are too technical for the non-technically trained person. One thing I never found was a complete discussion of kidney failure from a *patient's* point of view. This book aims to fill this void.

I realized early in the progression of my disease that I was ultimately responsible for my health and recovery. I felt that my doctors were my advisors, and that *I* was responsible for following their directions and for the decisions that we ultimately made. If I did not agree with a doctor or was unsure of what to do, I consulted with other doctors until I was convinced that a course of action was right for me. Realizing that you always have options to choose from, even if some of them are unattractive, gives you great power.

Before I started dialysis, my doctor had me complete a form outlining several dialysis treatment options. In addition to the two types of dialysis, the form gave me the choice of declining dialysis. Declining dialysis would have meant that I would die. Instead, I *chose* to live.

Having choices gives you control. One of the worst aspects of having a chronic disease is feeling helpless and not knowing what to do. Control can seem like merely telling people what to do. However, it is not that simple. Being in control comes from having knowledge of your condition and being able to articulate your views and pose questions to your doctors and others from a calm, informed perspective. Getting to the point of feeling in control can take time. Keeping an open mind to the possibilities of recovery can help you maintain a positive attitude toward your disease.

Once our kidneys fail, we have only two treatment choices: dialysis (either peritoneal dialysis or hemodialysis) or transplantation. A major issue for people with kidney failure is deciding which form of treatment is best. Often we will just accept what our doctors tell us without thinking much about how the treatment will change our lives. I was surprised at how little doctors knew about the day-to-day aspects of living with the treatments they prescribed. For me, it was important to make up my own mind and feel that I had control over what happened to me. I found that feeling in control (or even having the illusion of control) was the most helpful factor in facing kidney failure. Feeling in control may help you with your chronic illness.

In addition, researchers have discovered numerous ways, including using medications and following nutritional guidelines, either to prevent your kidneys from failing or to reduce the rate of their deterioration. Even if your kidneys eventually fail, there are approaches to making your life easier and more productive.

Coping Skills

When the reality of kidney failure set in, I was frightened and didn't know what to do. Over the decade during which my kidneys were failing and at the end of which I received a successful transplant, I learned how to manage my disease. Sometimes it wasn't easy. General information about kidney failure and treatment options was available, but information about *how* to decide which options to pursue and *how* to adapt to them were not. From my experience, I will share some considerations I had with my disease that I hope will help you with your own experience. First, here are some general coping skills I learned that helped me. They may help you, too.

Move Quickly through Denial and Face Your Disease Directly

I experienced all the emotional reactions to loss, described earlier, to varying degrees, but finally realized that I was ultimately responsible for my health. I had to accept that I was sick. Although the thought was unpleasant and I wanted to hide from it, in the final analysis, I was better off confronting my disease. No one would be more motivated than I would be to get well and live as well as I could. In a sense, I felt empowered by accepting my disease.

Be Your Own Advocate

In addition to educating myself about my disease to reduce fear, I found it important to use my knowledge to help my doctors give me the best care possible. Doctors cannot read minds. They often rely on feedback from their patients about how they feel and about reactions to treatments that they prescribe. If you do not tell your doctors about your reactions to their treatments, they will have a more difficult job in treating you. Furthermore, doctors should understand how these treatments affect your life. After all, *you* have to live with them. Do not be afraid to ask questions or challenge a treatment option if you think you cannot handle it. If you are too sick to be your own advocate, find someone who can do that for you. It can be a family member or friend. My friends helped me when my condition was very serious.

Doctors do their best to be aware of the latest treatments available for you. However, some new approach may come along that you might want to pursue. Discuss it with your doctor to determine if it might be beneficial for you. Be satisfied that you are receiving the best and most effective treatment for your disease.

Embrace Your Inner Strength

We have different personalities and temperaments. On one extreme, some people feel weak and powerless, sensing that they have little control over their lives. Mostly, they depend on others for support and feel that they cannot live without the help of others. At the other extreme, some people feel in total control and independent. They can take on the world and do things with help from relatively few people. Most of us fall between these two extremes.

When adversity strikes, even the strongest of us can question ourselves and doubt our ability to conquer our situation. The weakest can feel even more helpless and hopeless. I was in the middle. I went through many self-doubts when I knew my kidneys would fail. However, I discovered in time that I had a reserve of inner strength that I had not appreciated. To survive psychologically, I had to find that inner strength. I am not sure how I found it, but I think it came from a strong desire to survive. Once I knew I had this inner strength and realized I needed to improve my situation and conquer my disease largely alone, I embraced my strength. You, too, can do it. I have no secret formula, but you will find it, if you allow yourself to look for your inner strength and use it to help you through the difficult times. Some people turn to religion to find the strength, whereas others discover it in their ability to solve their own problems. No matter how you do it, I have learned that finding and embracing your inner strength is worth the journey.

Believe Your Life Will Improve

Having a chronic disease, especially kidney disease, does not necessarily mean that your life is over. It is amazing how people with the most debilitating diseases or injuries often go on to have fulfilling lives. Take, for example, the late Christopher Reeve, the actor who became quadriplegic after falling from a horse, breaking his neck, and severing his spinal cord. Despite his grave injuries, Reeve firmly believed that he would walk again. He faced his difficult circumstances with courage, dignity, and passion, and he became an effective advocate for increasing research funding to treat spinal cord injuries. Although he ultimately died from complications related to his injury, while he lived Reeve significantly raised awareness of spinal cord injury and helped increase research funding—accomplishments that must have been very gratifying to him.

In my own case, what kept me going was the belief that in the end, I would receive a transplant and my life would be better. I was discouraged from time to time, but I did not lose sight of the goal of receiving a new kidney. I even began planning activities I wanted to pursue, like traveling and flying airplanes.

Take the Long View

The mind has a way of blurring memories the longer time goes by. My memories of nasty hospital stays or major surgeries faded once I received my kidney transplant. Thus, when I confronted what appeared to be a difficult situation, I looked ahead to the point when my memory would be fuzzy. I believed everything would eventually be okay. When friends of mine face surgery or other traumatic events, I keep reminding them that in six months, their emotional responses will be considerably less intense than they are at the present.

Remain Optimistic and Give a Positive Spin to Everything

Often there were times when my situation seemed bleak. On a few occasions, there was the possibility that I might not survive. I found it extremely important to believe that I would get better. Although no specific cure was available for PKD, I knew that I could be treated successfully for kidney failure. Whether I remained on dialysis or received a transplant, I believed that I could create a fulfilling life. Regardless of what happened to me, I always tried to look at my situation with optimism. This made my recovery much easier.

Know Your Priorities and Stick to Them

As a kidney dialysis patient, I was continually fatigued, which limited my participation in many of the activities I enjoyed. Considering the competing demands that I confronted every day, I knew that I could not respond to everything. Instead, I developed a list of priorities that were important to me. My health was at the top of the list. Without my health, none of the other priorities mattered. Having priorities helped me decide what I could do or what I could not do. It was very important for me to learn the word "no." If a request was not consistent with my priorities, I did not feel obliged to accept.

Be Willing to Take Risks

Doctors are not always sure why their patients are sick. They can run a multitude of medical tests, and the cause of the illness still may not be clear. That happened to me when I developed a number of serious infections in 1999. At the time, I was on dialysis. During my many visits to the hospital, my doctors performed all types of procedures to locate the source of infection, but to no avail. Many patients with PKD have kidney infections, and medical tests may show some objective diagnostic measures to verify a diagnosis of kidney infection. For example, blood or urine cultures might have found evidence for bacteria. However, none of my cultures did.

Based on their experience, several nephrologists recommended that I have my kidneys removed. I was not particularly crazy about such a prospect, because I was still passing a fair amount of urine for a person with kidney failure, and having my kidneys removed was life-threatening, major surgery. However, I could not receive a transplant with an active infection or one suppressed by antibiotics. On the other hand, I could have my kidneys removed and still have the infections. I did not want to place myself at such risk for nothing. It was not a sure thing. But because I wanted a transplant, I felt that I had to take the risk and had both kidneys removed. Fortunately, everything worked out alright. The infections disappeared after the surgeon removed my kidneys, and over the succeeding months, I felt progressively better. The risk ultimately was worth it.

Ask for Help, But Don't Depend on It

When I was very sick I could not do some things on my own, like driving or shopping. Most of the time, I had friends who could help me when I needed it. However, they were not always available, especially on short notice. I found that it was important to have backup plans, like using taxis or county services for transportation or even a home worker if needed. Keep in mind that care-givers have lives and responsibilities of their own and may not have endless time and energy to devote to you. I found that if I worked to be independent, even when I felt at my worst, I avoided feeling helpless.

Keep Your Sense of Humor

Someone once said that laughter is the best medicine. I found that to be true in my case as well. Finding the humor in life's challenges can be freeing. For example, many of us in my dialysis center engaged in our own form of black humor. In a Frankensteinian sort of way, we would poke fun at all the tubes and gadgets that attached us to dialysis machines. Some people not familiar with dialysis did not understand the humor or were uncomfortable with it. That's okay—even beyond illness, life provides plenty of things to laugh about.

Our kidneys are involved in many of the amazing processes that help our bodies function. In the following chapter we'll take a closer look at the kidneys and how they work.

2

WHAT KIDNEYS DO

The kidney is an exceptionally sophisticated and efficient purification system that cleanses the blood of unwanted byproducts produced by the body. (These byproducts are called *metabolites*.) Although we have two kidneys, we need only one kidney to live. In fact, people can lose most of their kidney function without becoming ill.

Most organs in the body control only one function. The heart pumps blood, and the stomach digests food. But kidneys not only filter blood, they also regulate a number of other body functions:

- Balancing the amount of water and salts (called *electrolytes*) retained by the body
- Controlling blood pressure
- Maintaining the proper balance of acidity in the blood
- Regulating the production of red blood cells (called *erythrocytes*) that carry oxygen to the various organs of the body

- Controlling the level of phosphate in the blood
- Activating vitamin D

The kidneys function to keep conditions in the body within a normal range, known as *homeostasis*. All of these functions can be affected when kidneys fail.

Filtration

Humans are not the only animals with kidneys. All vertebrates (animals that have a spine) have kidneys. The earliest vertebrates lived in water. Because fish take a lot of water into their bodies, they need a mechanism to eliminate excess amounts. Saltwater fish also require a means to eliminate excess salt that they absorb. If saltwater fish could not expel excess water and salt from their bodies, they would blow up like a balloon and eventually explode. Kidneys may have evolved in animals to regulate water and salt balance.

Kidneys in vertebrates like us also eliminate waste products. Waste products are produced when we digest proteins (like those found in meat, fish, or dairy products). *Carbohydrates* (sugars and starches) are eventually broken down (metabolized) into water and *carbon dioxide*. However, when glucose (or sugar) exceeds a certain level in the blood, the kidney begins eliminating the excess. When a person's body expels sugar in the urine, it can be a sign that the person has diabetes (see chapter 3).

Kidneys are the body's simple filtration system. A simple system for filtering liquids removes particles that are greater than a certain size, whether they be coffee grounds or microbes. Filters usually have four parts: (1) a reservoir into which the liquid passes, like a funnel; (2) the filter itself, like porous paper, membranes, or cheesecloth; (3) the funnel stem, like a hose or straw; and (4) a collection receptacle, like a bottle or jar. We use filters every day when we percolate coffee or purify tap water. Most filtration systems use paper or activated charcoal as filters. Kidneys are a bit more complicated, but their filtration system works in a similar way.

The kidney is bean-shaped, approximately the size of an adult's fist, and weighs about half a pound. Like a simple filtration system, the kidney has four basic parts. Looking at figure 2.1, which compares the kidneys with a funnel, we see that blood containing wastes first enters the kidney from a branch of the renal artery, which is like the reservoir of the funnel. The blood passes through the filtration apparatus, called the *nephron*. Each kidney contains about one million nephrons. Nephrons are composed of the glomerulus, the tubular system, and the collecting duct.

The first part of the nephron is the *glomerulus* (the filter), which has a large surface area to provide efficient filtration. The larger or thicker the filter, the more efficiently it traps bigger particles. The glomerulus allows small molecules to pass through it while retaining large substances that the body needs, like various blood cells and protein molecules, and eliminates waste products the body does not need. In the kidney, filtration occurs as the blood is forced through the walls of the glomerulus and numerous small vessels, through which blood cells cannot pass, into the tubular system (the stem of the funnel). Filtration produces a plasma-like fluid called filtrate. Substances that the body still needs pass through the glomerulus.

The filtrate leaves the glomerulus and enters the tubules and collecting ducts, where the useful substances are reabsorbed. Unlike the hollow stem of a simple funnel, tubules and collecting ducts are highly complex, with specialized structures that remove waste products while reabsorbing nutrients and salts that the body

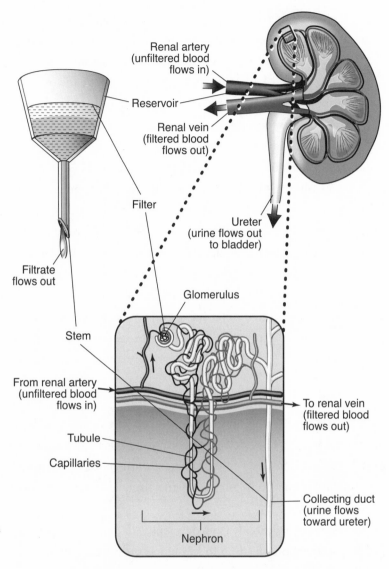

Figure 2.1. The Funneling Properties of the Kidney

needs. What is left is urine. The collecting duct connected to the bladder (the collection receptacle, akin to the coffee pot) provides the final filtration step for urine before the body eliminates it.

Let's take a closer look at the tubular system. As we see in figure 2.1, the tubules attach to the glomerulus and loop through the kidney. Tubules eliminate *urea*, the main byproduct of protein breakdown from the body. However, the body needs some of the salts, water, and other nutrients that also pass from the blood through the kidney's filter (glomerulus) into the filtrate. The tubules at various points on the loops process the filtrate further to reabsorb into the capillaries the salts, water, and nutrients the body needs back into the blood. Any excess salts and water not needed by the body remain in the filtrate to be eliminated as urine. So, the entire process of filtration that takes place in the kidneys involves filtering and reabsorbing—until everything useful has been reabsorbed and everything else is sent to the bladder to be eliminated from the body as urine.

Regulating Blood Pressure

In addition to filtering, kidneys help keep blood pressure from dropping too low. They do so by making and releasing an enzyme called *renin*. Maintaining blood pressure with renin involves several organs in the body, including the liver, lungs, and adrenal glands (see figure 2.2).

Renin prevents the body from developing dangerously low *sodium* (salt) concentrations, leading to low blood pressure. Such a condition can occur in hot weather, when the body sweats profusely, or with substantial blood loss. To prevent low blood pressure during salt depletion, the kidney releases renin into the bloodstream. When renin reaches the liver, it reacts with a protein called *angiotensinogen* to produce a biologically inactive protein called *angiotensin I*.

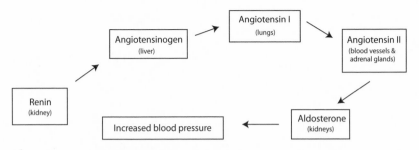

Figure 2.2. How Renin Regulates Blood Pressure

When angiotensin I leaves the liver, it travels to the lungs, where it is converted in the veins to *angiotensin II*. While traveling through the body, angiotensin II constricts blood vessels and raises blood pressure. In addition, angiotensin II acts on the *adrenal glands*, two small endocrine glands, one located on top of each kidney. In the adrenal gland, angiotensin II stimulates the release of the hormone called *aldosterone*, which can direct the kidneys to retain sodium and water. It's easy to see how the overproduction of renin can contribute to high blood pressure (see chapter 3).

Regulating Blood Acidity

The body maintains the blood's narrow range of acidity with buffers. The buffering process is regulated predominantly by a balance between carbonic acid and bicarbonate (baking soda) in the blood and by the acidity of the urine. In the kidney, acid along the tubular membrane swaps places with sodium (one of the salts) and bicarbonate. Various conditions can change the acidity of the blood. If you breathe too hard and too fast, the blood can become less acidic because of a reduction of carbon dioxide. If the kidney does not function properly, acid can accumulate, a condition known as *acidosis*.

Producing Red Blood Cells

Bone marrow makes red blood cells (erythrocytes) that carry oxygen throughout the body. Red blood cells live about four months and then must be replaced. The kidneys produce a hormone called *erythropoietin*, which controls the rate at which red blood cells form. When the kidney senses too little oxygen in the blood, it releases erythropoietin to stimulate the bone marrow to make more red blood cells. When kidney function is degraded or lost and the kidneys make insufficient erythropoietin, patients may have too few red blood cells, a condition called *anemia*.

Regulating Phosphate

Phosphate is essential for the body to produce energy. Dairy products are a major source of phosphate. Numerous chemical reactions in the body use phosphate, but our diets generally provide more phosphate than we need. The kidney is the only means of eliminating excess phosphate carried in the blood. If the kidney malfunctions, several problems can result from an excess of phosphate.

Phosphate readily combines with *calcium*. When excess phosphate binds to enough calcium, the body thinks it does not have enough calcium in the blood, prompting bones to release calcium into the bloodstream. When calcium is released into the bloodstream, people may develop *osteoporosis* and form calcium phosphate plaques in their organs, possibly leading to organ failure (see chapter 4).

Regulating Bone Structure

Excess phosphate in the blood is not the only cause of bone demineralization. *Vitamin D,* a fat-soluble vitamin, plays an important role in the body's absorption of calcium to maintain strong bones and

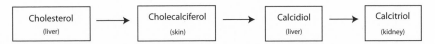

Figure 2.3. How Vitamin D Is Produced

teeth. Making vitamin D is a complicated process involving active and less active forms of vitamin D (see figure 2.3).

The body makes active forms of vitamin D from cholesterol. One way is from sunlight: ultraviolet light stimulates the formation of *cholecalciferol*, a derivative of cholesterol, in the skin. Activated cholecalciferol then passes through the liver and becomes an even more active form of vitamin D called *calcidiol*. The final activation of vitamin D occurs in the kidney. When calcidiol enters the kidney, it is converted to *calcitriol*, the only form of vitamin D that the body actually uses. Some dietary supplements contain cholecalciferol, bypassing the need for the sun's activation of less active forms of vitamin D. Failing kidneys may affect the body's ability to absorb vitamin D, which can lead to bone loss.

Many of the body's essential activities depend on normal kidney function. When kidneys fail, there are major consequences for the body. In the following chapter we discuss why kidneys may fail.

3

WHY KIDNEYS FAIL

Numerous health problems can lead to kidney failure. The four main causes are diabetes, hypertension, glomerular diseases, and polycystic kidney disease (PKD). Genetics plays a role in most causes of kidney failure, and kidney failure may result from a specific defect inherited from one or both parents. PKD is primarily an inherited kidney disease.

Genetics is not the whole story, however. Lifestyle and other environmental factors may also be significant influences. This chapter begins with a primer on the genetic and environmental factors contributing to kidney failure. Knowledge of these factors will help you understand how you might slow the progression of your disease.

Nature versus Nurture
Genetic Factors

All of the functions in our bodies operate on the basis of instructions embedded in our genetic code. Over the past fifty years, researchers have uncovered the intricate details of how this genetic code works. The Human Genome Project, which was completed in 2003, determined the complete nucleotide sequence of human *deoxyribonucleic acid* (DNA).

Genes provide a blueprint for creating our bodies and making them work. Just as the blueprints for a house show how to build its various parts, like the foundation, walls, and roof, genes direct the construction of cells, organs, bone, and skin. Moreover, like the heating, air conditioning, and electrical systems that control the environmental conditions in a house, genes control how our bodies function.

The primary purpose of genes is making *proteins*. Proteins are like a building's construction workers and engineers. They make and operate the human body according to the genetic blueprints residing within the *chromosomes*.

For all organs of the body, our genes issue the instructions (or blueprints) to make proteins while we are in the womb. For organs to develop correctly, certain processes must happen in an exact way. It starts when a sperm fertilizes the egg. The cells in the resulting embryo, possessing two copies of each gene, one from each parent, begin to divide. As the embryo grows, copies of genes inherited from each parent must be reproduced identically in each new cell, so that all the cells in the developing fetus (and eventually in the person's body) will have the same set of genetic blueprints. During a person's lifetime, many of the cells in the body will die and be replaced with new ones. These new cells generally also contain the same blueprints.

Although rare, mistakes can occur when genes are copied. Called *mutations*, these mistakes can cause the organs to work improperly. If a house's blueprints are wrong, a door might be located in the wrong place or the lighting system might fail because of incorrect wiring. In people, gene mistakes are passed along to their children and can cause them to inherit a disease. For example, mutations in genes that make or control kidneys can malfunction, leading to disease.

Environmental Factors

Behavioral and environmental factors can also contribute to the expression or progression of a disease. In the case of kidney failure, an improper diet and lack of exercise or other lifestyle factors can contribute greatly to a person's medical status. We do not deliberately set out to make ourselves ill. However, with the stresses of our culture and everyday life, it can be easy to neglect our own health. Between work, family, and social obligations, we are so busy that we may have little time to eat properly or to get adequate exercise. Over time, our health can begin to fail without our even knowing it.

When people don't eat right and don't exercise, they are more likely to be overweight or obese. Obesity has reached epidemic proportions in the United States and in other developed countries. According to a recent study, 66.3 percent of Americans are overweight, obese, or morbidly obese.[1] African Americans and Hispanic Americans have a higher prevalence of obesity than non-Hispanic whites. Moreover, women across all races are more obese than men. Obesity increases with age, leveling off by age 60 or declining thereafter.

Obesity may lead to other health complications—including kidney failure—because obesity makes people more likely to develop diabetes and hypertension. Excess weight can also cause coronary heart disease, high cholesterol levels, and stroke, which can lead to death.

Diseases That Cause Kidney Failure

References to the symptoms of kidney disorders by the ancient Greeks suggest that we have known about kidney failure for thousands of years. We weren't able to analyze kidneys and other organs until the nineteenth century, however. In 1827, the English physician Richard Bright first described the symptoms of kidney failure.

In the twenty-first century, kidney failure is still incurable, but it can be prevented and treated. With dialysis and transplantation, people with kidney failure can continue to have productive lives. Nevertheless, failing kidneys take a very high medical, emotional, and financial toll. There is no cure for kidney failure, but knowing its causes can help prevent, delay, or prepare for it.

As we learned in chapter 1, approximately one-half million people in the United States are living with kidney failure. In most cases, diabetes and hypertension are the causes. Both are preventable (see chapter 5). Glomerular disorders, which can have both environmental and genetic origins, are another cause of kidney failure. There are also inherited causes of kidney failure, like PKD. If a person inherits mutated genes, the disease will develop, although the progression of the disease varies among families and individuals. This chapter presents a brief overview of each of these four leading causes of kidney failure.

Diabetes

Diabetes (also known as diabetes mellitus) is the leading cause of kidney failure in the United States and accounts for 38 percent of cases. Because of rising obesity rates, diabetes rates are increasing, even among children. As many as 20.6 million people have diabetes. As people age, they become more susceptible to diabetes (see figure 3.1). About one-half of all people with diabetes are over 60

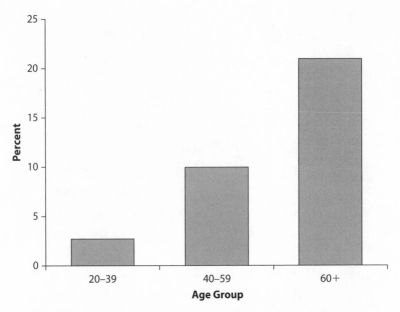

Figure 3.1. Estimated Total Prevalence of Diabetes in People Aged 20 Years and Older, by Age Group, United States, 2005

Source: 1999–2002 National Health and Nutrition Examination Survey estimates of total prevalence (both diagnosed and undiagnosed were projected to year 2005).

years old. Across the population, slightly more men than women have diabetes, and it disproportionately affects Native Americans, non-Hispanic African Americans, and Hispanic Americans (see figure 3.2). Understanding the underlying causes of diabetes is essential for learning how to prevent and treat it.

Diabetes is a metabolic disease in which the body does not properly utilize glucose. *Glucose* is the main source of energy in the body. In order for glucose to enter cells and produce energy, the pancreas secretes the protein *insulin* into the bloodstream to help glucose cross the membranes surrounding cells. If this process is interrupted, glucose accumulates in the blood and can spill out

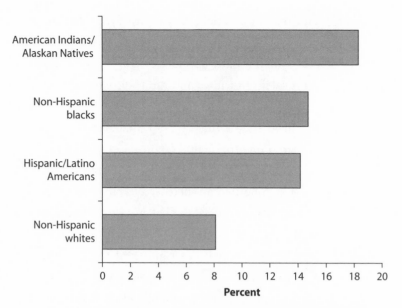

Figure 3.2. Estimated Age-Adjusted Total Prevalence of Diabetes in People Aged 20 Years and Older, by Race/Ethnicity, United States, 2005

Source: For American Indians/Alaskan Natives, the estimate of total prevalence was calculated using the estimate of diagnosed diabetes from the 2003 outpatient database of the Indian Health Service and the estimate of undiagnosed diabetes from the 1999–2002 National Health and Nutrition Examination Survey. For the other groups, 1999–2002 NHANES estimates of total prevalence (both diagnosed and undiagnosed) were projected to year 2005.

into the urine. Cells can starve without glucose, even with high concentrations of glucose in the blood, if it cannot permeate cell membranes.

The inability of insulin to process glucose efficiently can occur for one of two reasons: (1) a lack of sufficient insulin secretion by the pancreas or (2) a body's resistance to insulin, preventing the transport of glucose into the cells. When the pancreas does not secrete enough insulin, this condition is known as Type 1 diabetes. Attacks from the body's own immune system destroy beta cells, thereby reducing insulin secretion. People with Type I diabetes must take insulin to live. Five to 10 percent of people with diabetes have Type I diabetes, which usually develops in childhood. Type I diabetes is more prevalent in whites and rarely develops in people of other races.

Researchers have found that Type I diabetes develops because of genetic and environmental factors. Up to 50 percent of people with Type I diabetes have the disease because of genetic susceptibility—they inherited an increased likelihood of developing it. Mutations in a number of genes that encode proteins involved in the immune system play a significant role in the development of diabetes. Scientists believe that environmental triggers like viral infections, dietary factors, environmental toxins, psychological stress, and even season of the year can precipitate Type I diabetes. However, no single trigger appears responsible.

Type 2 diabetes, the number one cause of kidney failure, accounts for most cases of diabetes and is clearly linked to obesity. According to the National Institutes of Health, almost 80 percent of people with Type 2 diabetes are overweight.[2] In Type 2 diabetes, although the pancreas secretes plenty of insulin, the cells of the body become resistant to it, preventing the transport of glucose into the cells. Like people with Type I diabetes, people with Type 2 diabetes also may need insulin supplementation in order to live. Mild cases of Type 2 diabetes can be controlled through diet and oral, non-insulin medications.

Type 2 diabetes is much more prevalent in minority populations, largely because these groups have higher rates of obesity. Native Americans have one of the highest rates of Type 2 diabetes in the world. Other minority groups greatly affected by Type 2 diabetes include African Americans, non-Hispanic African Americans, and Hispanic Americans. Because of the high rates of obesity in these populations, the U.S. Centers for Disease Control and Prevention expects the rates of diabetes to increase in the future.

Diabetes can create many complications affecting almost every part of the body. In addition to kidney failure, diabetes can lead to heart and blood vessel disease, strokes, blindness, limb amputations, and nerve damage. Babies born to women with uncontrolled diabetes can have birth defects. This is all a big price to pay for a disease that is preventable in most cases by maintaining a normal weight. Medical researchers are working hard to identify the hormonal and environmental causes of increasing rates of obesity, and to develop treatments and programs to conquer the obesity epidemic. (See below for more information about hormones and obesity and about obesity and diabetes.)

Type 2 diabetes has a poorly understood genetic component. Research is under way to determine which genes are involved and to what extent they play a role in the development of the disease. Having answers to these questions will help doctors identify who is most susceptible to diabetes and locate potential targets for treatment.

Type 2 diabetes runs in families. However, the genetic basis of the mutations that lead to diabetes varies among family members. Thus, a number of different genes may be responsible for an increased susceptibility to Type 2 diabetes. Although researchers have studied so-called *polygenetic diseases* for more than twenty years, they have learned that finding the genes that contribute the most to a disease is quite difficult. Type 2 diabetes is no exception, especially considering the importance of environment and lifestyle in the disease. This does not mean that scientific research has yielded no new information about the genetic contribution to diabetes. Quite the contrary! Researchers have made a good start in identifying the genes involved.

Recently, three international genetic studies examined the genes involved in insulin secretion from pancreatic cells as well as how insulin acts on cells in the body.[3] These studies found at least ten genetic variants in diabetic populations, each one of which contributes small amounts to the predisposition for the disease. It is not known whether any of these variants suggest a novel approach to treating Type 2 diabetes. More extensive research is required.

Understanding the relationship between obesity and Type 2 diabetes is critical. The key to this relationship are the cells in the body and, interestingly, in the brain. Over the past decade, researchers have learned a great deal about the variety of substances that control appetite, including hormones.[4]

Hormones act on receptors to exert their functions. One of these functions is appetite. *Receptors* are specialized entities on surfaces of cell membranes that act specifically for only one hormone, similarly structured hormones, or synthetic compounds. Think of the hormone-receptor interaction as a key and a lock. Only one key (or keys very similar to it) will unlock the door so the hormone will respond appropriately.

One such hormone, called *leptin*, regulates appetite through an interaction with a receptor. Researchers have found that when blood leptin levels are high, we eat less, and when they are low, we eat more. When we eat, leptin levels increase. The ability of this hormone to tell us when we are full depends on its action on certain receptors, however. If these receptors do not respond appropriately to leptin, a person can eat more food despite being full, and obesity can result. Obese people often have higher leptin levels, which correlate with *insulin resistance*. The receptors may respond less to a given amount of leptin, and the body then secretes more of it. Exactly how changes in leptin levels, other proteins, and even inflammatory responses cause or relate to insulin resistance and diabetes is not known. However, the study of leptin levels is a promising area for future diabetes research.[5]

Another factor in insulin resistance resides in the brain. The brain regulates food intake by responding to levels of insulin and leptin in the blood, as well as to glucose and certain types of fat called free fatty acids. When the brain detects that the actions of these hormones are sufficient, it tells the rest of the body that it needs to consume less food. Conversely, when these signals are in short supply, the brain promotes increased food consumption. If the brain can no longer keep food intake within normal limits, weight gain and insulin resistance can result. How does this happen?

It turns out that the brain has insulin receptors that can become resistant to insulin, just as insulin receptors in peripheral tissues can. In fact, the biochemical pathways that mediate the actions of insulin appear to be similar in both the brain and peripheral tissues. Like peripheral tissues, the brain receptors become more resistant to insulin with excess food consumption. Thus, the brain's control of food intake is impaired, resulting in obesity. The brain responds to leptin in the same way as tissues do elsewhere in the body. How obesity can lead to Type 2 diabetes is a multifaceted process.

So, how does all this add up? When we eat, food is partially converted into glucose to feed the body's cells and to provide the energy they need to operate. To transport glucose into the cells, the pancreas secretes insulin, thereby regulating our blood levels of glucose. If we eat too much food over a long period, the cells, including those in the brain, become resistant to the constant bombardment of too much insulin. In addition, the release of leptin to control our food intake no longer controls our appetite, and we develop resistance to leptin. Finally, when insulin production is insufficient to move glucose into cells, glucose rises to dangerous levels in the blood and can result in Type 2 diabetes.

We have seen that there are many physiological mechanisms that can lead to obesity and diabetes. Genetic defects, too, can contribute to the ultimate expression of Type 2 diabetes. When these genes have been identified, it is likely that medications can be developed that will target the expression of these genes, potentially controlling excessive food intake.

How does diabetes lead to kidney failure? The process, technically known as *diabetic nephropathy*, typically develops over a period of ten to twenty-five years. It starts when excess glucose in the blood degrades the filtering capacity of the glomerulus in the kidney (see chapter 2). Normally, the glomerulus will allow only small molecules, like water and salts, to pass through, leaving behind large molecules like proteins. Small amounts of protein excreted in the urine, a condition called *microalbuminuria*, is often the first sign of diabetes. (A *sign* is something a doctor can identify through testing. A *symptom* is something the patient experiences or notices.) Kidney function is generally normal at this stage. However, if the deterioration of the filtration of blood through the glomerulus continues, increasing amounts of protein pass into the urine. Called *macroalbuminuria*, this excess excretion of protein can cause scarring of the glomerulus and can lead to declining kidney function.

How high glucose concentrations degrade kidney function is not completely understood. Nevertheless, researchers have discovered a number of potential biochemical pathways that are stimulated by glucose.[6] These pathways seem to underlie the growth of some cells in the glomerulus and tubules that lead to scarring and fiber-like tissue, thereby degrading kidney function. If these processes continue long enough, kidney failure can result.

Hypertension

Hypertension, or high blood pressure, is the second leading cause of kidney failure, accounting for 24 percent of cases. Blood pressure that is too high can damage kidneys and cause them to ultimately fail. (High blood pressure is defined below.)

When the heart pumps blood through the blood vessels, the blood pushing against the walls of these vessels increases the pressure. Two numbers express this pressure: one is pressure when the heart has contracted (known as maximum, or systolic, pressure), and the other is the pressure after the heart relaxes (known as minimum, or diastolic, pressure).

Blood pressure can be measured using a blood pressure monitor. A blood pressure cuff is wrapped around the upper arm. The cuff is inflated using a pump until the pulse in the upper arm is no longer felt. The cuff is slowly deflated until the sounds of heartbeats are heard. The pressure at which the sounds are first heard is the systolic pressure, whereas the pressure at which sounds are no longer detectable is the diastolic pressure. The blood pressure monitor provides a readout of two numbers. The measured blood pressure is expressed as a ratio of these two numbers, like 120/80 (systolic/diastolic, or "systolic over diastolic").

A blood pressure at or below 120/80 is considered normal. Higher values may be evidence of high blood pressure, or *hypertension*. Hypertension is categorized as more or less severe based on the degree of pressure elevation. According to the National Institutes of Health, if the systolic pressure reaches 120 to 139 or the diastolic pressure reaches 80 to 89, a person is pre-hypertensive. People with systolic pressures of 140 and above, or diastolic pressures of 90 or above, are considered hypertensive. In either case, medications and/or lifestyle changes are necessary to control blood pressure.

As we see in figure 3.3, two factors contribute to the development of hypertension: the amount of blood flowing through vessels
and the vessels' diameter. These factors affect either the systolic or
the diastolic pressures. The amount of blood flowing through
blood vessels results from the volume of blood leaving the heart
with each contraction and the heart rate. The higher the volume of
blood expelled or the higher the heart rate, the higher the systolic
blood pressure. The diameter of the blood vessels affects blood

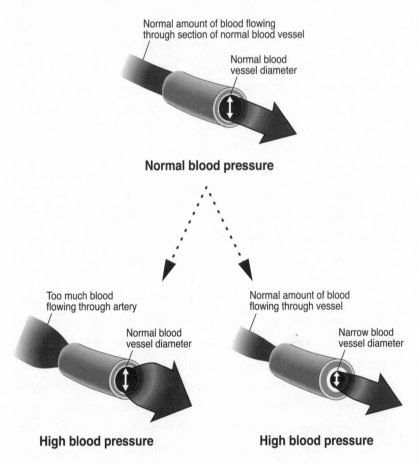

Figure 3.3. Factors in High Blood Pressure

pressure by resisting blood flow. The smaller the diameter of the vessels, the higher the diastolic blood pressure. This is analogous to putting your thumb over the tip of a hose with running water. Constricting the hose nozzle with your thumb, you can feel the water pressure build. One reason that vessels may be small is because of blockages due to *atherosclerosis* (a buildup of plaque within the vessels). There are other reasons, like other underlying medical problems, and appropriate medical treatment is determined by the cause of hypertension (see chapter 5).

Blood pressure is not just influenced by physiological factors like varying heart rates and the muscular tone of blood vessels. Genetic susceptibility may also influence a person's blood pressure. Just as in diabetes research, determining which specific genes are responsible for blood pressure and their relative contribution to hypertension has been very difficult.[7] Researchers do not expect that a mutation in a single gene is responsible for hypertension. Most likely, the interplay of many genes promotes hypertension. Environment and lifestyle can also contribute to hypertension through a complex gene-environment interaction. One example of this type of interaction is excessive salt (sodium) intake and retention.

Excess salt intake can lead to hypertension. However, each person responds to salt differently. At the extremes, some people are very sensitive to salt, whereas some are insensitive. These differences suggest that salt sensitivity has a genetic component. As we learned in chapter 2, the renin-angiotensin system evolved to combat dehydration by retaining sodium and maintaining blood pressure when the body loses sodium. In this system alone, it is possible that many genes could be altered in a way that promotes hypertension.

Research on genes underlying hypertension is still in its infancy and will require many more studies to identify the specific genes responsible. Future research may also yield new medications to reduce hypertension. Because hypertension plays such an important role in kidney disease, these new medications may give physicians better tools to prevent kidney failure.

Obesity contributes to hypertension as well as kidney damage induced by other diseases discussed in this chapter. Kidney diseases themselves are associated with increased blood pressure by a variety of mechanisms. Obese people often take in an excessive amount of salt, which can lead to hypertension. The high pressure on the glomerulus can slowly degrade its filtering capacity and precipitate reactions similar to those that occur in diabetes-induced kidney failure. In addition, accumulating fat can contribute to hypertension. Considering that obesity, hypertension, and diabetes often accompany one another, it is hard to know which problem came first. However, obesity is often the primary cause of hypertension and diabetes.

We know that hypertension slowly destroys the kidneys' ability to filter the blood, but how does hypertension lead to kidney failure? With prolonged hypertension, the excess pressure can injure small blood vessels in the kidney and can destroy the filtering ability of the glomerulus (see chapter 2), leading to kidney failure. Using the hose metaphor, if you attach cheesecloth tightly over the end of the hose, water will flow through the cheesecloth without harming it. But if you pinch the hose, increasing the flow pressure, the cheesecloth will begin to degrade and eventually rupture.

Glomerular Diseases

Glomerular diseases are a complex set of disorders and are the third leading cause of kidney failure in the United States, accounting for 15 percent of cases. Glomerular disease often results in inflammation of the glomerulus, which can eventually cause the formation of scar tissue. As a result, protein leaks into the urine instead of being absorbed back into circulation. Like diabetes and hypertension, glomerular diseases slowly destroy the filtering ability of the glomerulus. Excess pressure on the sensitive glomerulus can lead to kidney failure. The three main causes of glomerular diseases are autoimmune diseases, hereditary nephritis, and infections.

The body's immune system provides the first line of defense against infections by generating antibodies and immunoglobulins. However, there are times when antibodies and immunoglobulins cause harm to the body, which can lead to a number of medical problems. One of these complications is the deposit of antibodies in the glomeruli, causing inflammation.

Many autoimmune disorders contribute to glomerular diseases. One of these diseases is immunoglobulin A (IgA) nephropathy. IgA nephropathy is the most common cause of glomerular diseases not related to the presence of another disease. With IgA nephropathy, IgA deposits on the glomerulus, causing inflammation. IgA nephropathy affects men and women of all age groups equally. When a considerable amount of protein appears in the urine, controlling blood pressure helps manage the symptoms and may slow the rate of deterioration of kidney function.

Lupus erythematosus, another autoimmune disease, primarily involves inflammation of the skin and joints. This disease affects more women than men. When lupus erythematosus attacks the kidney, autoantibodies form or are deposited in the glomeruli and cause scarring. Drugs that suppress the immune system are generally used to treat the inflammation in the kidney.

One inherited form of glomerular diseases is Alport syndrome. Alport syndrome not only affects the kidney but may also impair vision and hearing. More men have difficulty with this disease than women, experiencing a decline in kidney function in their twenties and reaching total kidney failure by age 40.

Glomerular diseases are also caused by infections in other parts of the body. Similar to what happens in autoimmune diseases, the high number of antibodies produced to combat these infections can deposit in the kidneys and reduce kidney function. Although infections usually do not cause permanent damage, people with chronic infectious diseases like HIV/AIDS and hepatitis C have a risk of developing chronic kidney failure.

Focal segmental glomerulosclerosis is another glomerular disease that disproportionately affects African Americans. It results in scarring of the glomerulus or clustering of glomeruli in a specific segment of the kidney. Focal segmental glomerulosclerosis can be difficult to diagnose and treat. Biopsies to search for scarring in kidney tissue are the best means of a diagnosis. (A *biopsy* is a procedure in which a small amount of tissue is removed from the body for investigation and testing.) However, if the biopsy sample is from an unaffected area of the kidney, scarring will not be evident. Thus, repeated biopsies in different segments of the kidney are needed to confirm a diagnosis of focal segmental glomerulosclerosis.

Polycystic Kidney Disease

Polycystic kidney disease (PKD), the fourth leading cause of kidney failure, accounts for about 5 percent of people with kidney failure. In PKD, small, fluid-filled cysts develop in the kidneys, sometimes even before birth. These cysts grow large enough over time to cause kidney failure. Because the cysts can grow so large, physicians used to think PKD was a form of kidney cancer.

According to the PKD Foundation, PKD affects 600,000 Americans of both genders and all ethnic groups. PKD has the strongest genetic link to a kidney disease. Although it can occur spontaneously, most people get PKD by inheriting it. In fact, PKD is one of the most life-threatening inherited diseases. Because PKD is primarily inherited, research has identified the genes and their corresponding proteins. As a result, a cure for PKD may be found in the near future.

People with PKD inherit the disease from one or both of their parents, depending on the form of the disease. PKD comes in two forms: *autosomal dominant (ADPKD)*, the more common form of the disease, and *autosomal recessive (ARPKD)*.

Genetically, the difference between ADPKD and ARPKD is the number of faulty copies inherited (see figures 3.4 and 3.5). People with ADPKD inherit the mutated gene from only one parent, whereas people with ARPKD inherit one mutated gene from both parents. The gene inherited in ARPKD is different from the one inherited in ADPKD.

ADPKD is very common, affecting 1 in 500 people. Because a person needs to inherit only one copy of an abnormal gene from one affected parent to get ADPKD, the chance of inheriting PKD when one parent has the defect is 50 percent. Because both parents must have the mutated gene, inheriting ARPKD is much less common, affecting 1 in 20,000 people in the general population. With ARPKD, if only one parent carries the mutated gene without having the disease himself, children will not develop ARPKD but may pass on the mutated gene to their children. A person with parents who both have a mutated ARPKD gene has only a 25 percent chance of inheriting the disease.

ADPKD and ARPKD also develop differently. The onset of ADPKD can occur at any age from the late teens to the mid-thirties, with kidney failure generally developing between the mid-forties and mid-fifties. Because the rate of cyst formation is variable, a person with ADPKD may not need dialysis until an advanced age. Sometimes ADPKD is diagnosed unexpectedly during a routine

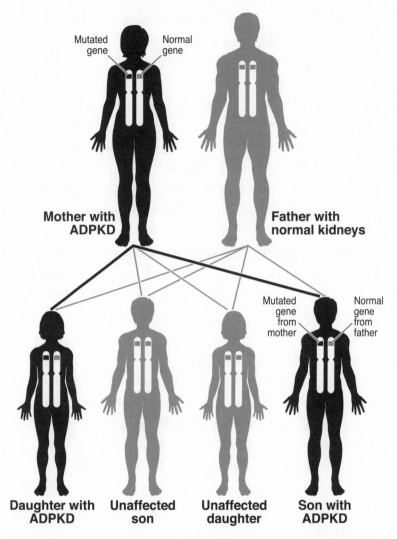

Figure 3.4. Autosomal Dominant Inheritance of PKD (ADPKD)

physical, where abnormal lab results suggest kidney disease. More tests would be needed for a definitive diagnosis (see below). ARPKD, in comparison, often progresses before birth. A person with ARPKD can only survive into adulthood with dialysis or

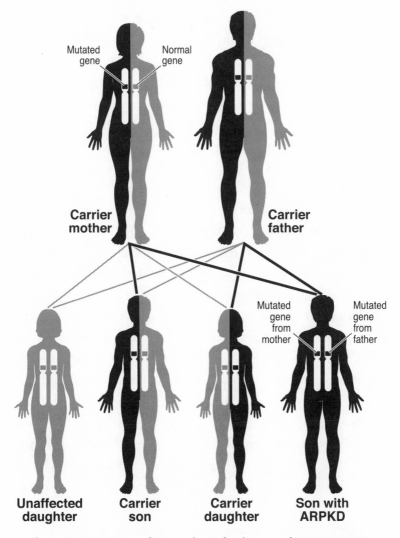

Figure 3.5. Autosomal Recessive Inheritance of PKD (ARPKD)

transplantation. In this book I use the terms ADPKD and PKD interchangeably, since the incidence of ARPKD is so low.

During the last decade research has revealed the genetic underpinnings of PKD. Two genes, *PKD1* and *PKD2*, account for virtually all cases of PKD. Mutations in *PKD1* account for 85 percent of PKD cases. In most of the other cases of PKD, mutations in *PKD2* are responsible.

Although the disease caused by each mutated gene is similar, people with *PKD2* mutations tend to progress toward kidney failure later in life than people with *PKD1* mutations. In addition, people with *PKD2* mutations have fewer renal cysts when diagnosed and are less likely to have high blood pressure. People with *PKD1* mutations experience kidney failure earlier in life because they have more cysts than people with *PKD2* mutations.

Genes make proteins. *PKD1* and *PKD2* make the proteins polycystin-1 and polycystin-2, respectively, which play a crucial role in the growth of cysts, though we don't yet know exactly how. Research has shown that the two proteins are attached to one another and that mutations in either gene can cause PKD. Although a mutation in the genes and improper working of the proteins are necessary for PKD to progress, other unknown factors may explain why the disease develops differently across families and even within families.

How renal cysts form and grow is currently under intense scientific investigation. Epithelial cells lining the tubules in the kidneys are actively involved in reabsorbing nutrients and water (see chapter 2). In PKD, 1 to 2 percent of epithelial cells reproduce many times and eventually form numerous cysts. These cysts fill up with fluid and eventually press against the nephrons so that no urine can pass through them. When enough nephrons are blocked, the kidneys cease to function. The cysts that form in the kidneys can become quite large (see figure 3.6). A normal kidney weighs less than a pound. A polycystic kidney can weigh up to 38 pounds and may produce a protruding abdomen.

Until recently, early diagnosis of PKD had been difficult, but now non-invasive techniques like ultrasound, computerized tomography

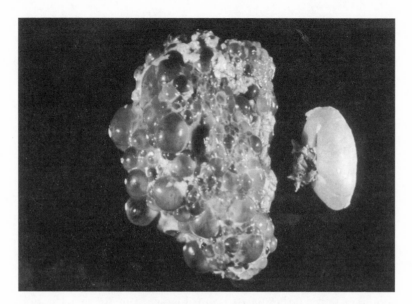

Figure 3.6. A Polycystic Kidney *(left)* Can Be Much Larger Than a Normal Kidney *(right)*

Source: PKD Foundation.

(CT) scans, and magnetic resonance imaging (MRI) scans are used to identify renal cysts.[8] Ultrasound detects ADPKD in most people by 30 years of age. However, ultrasound may miss some cases involving the *PKD2* gene. CT scans produce clearer images but require exposure to radiation and contrast dyes.

A recent study found that measuring increases in kidney size (cyst volume) using MRI scans is the best method of diagnosing and following the progression of PKD, and was an excellent predictor of the loss of kidney function.[9] Using MRI scans to measure kidney size is not yet part of general clinical practice, but this approach could provide more precise measurements of disease progression and of the effectiveness of medical treatments.

Like diabetes, PKD can have numerous health consequences. Kidney cysts can be quite painful and may require surgery. People with PKD may have blood in the urine, frequent kidney infections, and urinary tract infections that require hospitalization. In some cases, the kidneys must be removed.

People with PKD may also have cysts form in the liver or other organs. The cysts can become large and uncomfortable, especially in women, requiring removal of part of the liver or drainage of the fluid in the cysts.

A potentially fatal complication of PKD is the ballooning (called an *aneurysm*) and rupture of a major blood vessel, especially in the brain. Aneurysms occur in 5 to 10 percent of people with PKD. Where a family history of aneurysms exists, the risk of aneurysm rises to 20 percent. Modern imaging techniques can detect aneurysms by visualizing affected blood vessels, and people with PKD should be tested if they have a family history of aneurysms. If found early, aneurysms of a certain size can be repaired surgically. Small aneurysms are monitored with periodic scans.

Genetic Tests

Because genetic influences contribute to all four causes of kidney failure we have discussed, can tests identify people who are (or whose descendents are) at risk of developing kidney disease? Would a test help these people modify their lifestyle to reduce their chances of getting kidney disease or developing kidney failure? Perhaps. Some genetic tests can find the genes that cause diseases like diabetes. But because so many genes can contribute to each disease, it is not clear at this time how valuable such tests would be.

PKD is an exception because the genes for the disease have been identified. A genetic test has been developed by Athena Diagnostics (www.renaldx.com) to sequence *PKD1* and *PKD2* and to look for mutations. The test is effective only 70 percent of the time, however, so the results are possibly misleading. Sometimes the results give a false positive for the presence of PKD. Conversely, the results can miss actual cases of PKD. Results of these genetic tests should be confirmed by an ultrasound.

Although genetic testing has its advantages, there are disadvantages that might deter some people from being tested. One drawback of finding out you have a disease is the emotional burden that knowledge brings with it. Since there is little you can do about having PKD, other than good medical management for symptoms like hypertension and drinking a lot of fluid, what purpose would be served by knowing? A diagnosis of PKD may make it difficult to obtain medical and life insurance. If you do not have continuous employment as I did, a new employer may not provide adequate insurance. If you are unemployed, you may not be able to obtain insurance at all. Having a definitive diagnosis of PKD may not be useful until signs of kidney failure or other symptoms like hypertension or kidney cysts appear. Recently legislation to bar genetic discrimination in obtaining medical insurance and employment was signed into federal law, the Genetic Information Non-Discrimination Act of 2008. Currently it is not clear how well the law will be enforced or whether it will face legal challenges. In addition, Congress passed the Patient Protection and Affordable Care Act in 2010 that prohibits excluding people with preexisting conditions from obtaining health insurance by 2014.

People with PKD may have trouble deciding whether to have children. Although children have a 50-50 chance of *not* inheriting a PKD mutated gene from an affected parent, they also have a 50-50 chance of inheriting the disease. These odds are high enough to give some people pause before deciding to start a family. Parents can take solace in the hope that a cure might emerge for their children with PKD. In my own family, my mother died prematurely at age 44, when dialysis and transplantation were not available. Now in my sixties, I have survived with a successful kidney transplant and am living a normal life. Today's medicine can treat kidney failure, anemia, high blood pressure, and other complicating factors of the disease. In my mother's day, none of these treatments existed. Tomorrow's medicine may be much more advanced, and a treatment to prevent cyst formation or growth may be available, relieving our children of the burden of PKD.

There is hope for better treatment options in the future.

4

DIAGNOSING AND
MANAGING KIDNEY DISEASE

E very person should get a checkup with a primary care physician at least once a year. It may be while you are having one of these annual checkups that your doctor discovers that you are at risk for kidney disease or that you already have kidney disease. Although kidney disease usually has no symptoms, like fatigue or pain, a physical examination can determine whether you have high blood pressure, blood in the urine, or decreased kidney function. A thorough medical history helps your doctor know whether you have a predisposition to kidney disease or a family history of diseases that can lead to kidney disease, like diabetes, high blood pressure, or polycystic kidney disease (PKD).

If you have one or more of these risk factors, your doctor may order additional screening tests. The National Kidney Foundation (NKF) has developed a screening program for risk of developing kidney disease called the Kidney Early Evaluation Program (KEEP).

Your doctor may use certain measures to assess your risk and to find any evidence of kidney disease and whether it has progressed. Table 4.1 lists the measures of assessing risk. Screening typically consists of *urinalysis* (looking for protein or blood in the urine) and measuring creatinine or other factors in the blood. With a measure of blood creatinine, your doctor will calculate your glomerular filtration rate, a measure of the ability of your kidneys to filter toxins from your blood. The results of these tests may cause your doctor to suspect that you have kidney disease. A definite plus is that the results of the tests may provide an early warning, so your doctor can help you protect your kidneys from further damage and educate you about treatment options or changes in lifestyle. For example, your doctor may recommend that you lose weight, stop smoking, or control your blood pressure.

Table 4.1
Kidney Early Evaluation Program (KEEP) Screening Measures

Measures	Significance
↑ Blood pressure	Risk of kidney disease
Height, weight, and waist circumference	Obesity; risk of diabetes and kidney disease
↑ Blood glucose	Risk of diabetes
↓ Hemoglobin	Anemia
White blood cells in urine	Risk for infections, inflammation, and other abnormalities in the urinary tract
Red blood cells in the urine	Evidence of kidney disease
Protein in the urine	Evidence of kidney disease
↓ Glomerular filtration rate	Evidence of kidney failure
↑ Total cholesterol, ↓ HDL, ↑ LDL, and ↑ triglycerides	Risk for cardiovascular disease
↓ Calcium, ↑ phosphorus, ↑ parathyroid hormone	Evidence of possible bone disease

Source: Adapted from the list of KEEP measures from National Kidney Foundation website at www.kidney.org.

Being diagnosed with any disease can be terrifying. If you are diagnosed with kidney disease, gather as much information as you can about your condition and medical care, find ways to reduce the progression of kidney disease, and plan your future. Take an active role in your care. It will go a long way toward helping you feel more in control. This chapter covers some of the diagnostic tools and treatments involved with your medical care.

Diagnostics

Doctors monitor kidney function in their patients by measuring substances in the blood and urine using several laboratory tests: blood urea nitrogen (BUN), or just urea, creatinine, creatinine clearance, and glomerular filtration rate (GFR). To perform these tests, your health care provider will draw small amounts of blood and will ask you for a urine sample.

Urea and creatinine in the blood are measures of the main products of protein metabolism. How concentrated these substances are in the blood indicates how effectively your kidneys remove waste products. Normal concentrations of these substances are 15 to 25 mg/dl for BUN and 0.5 to 1.3 mg/dl for creatinine (mg/dl [milligrams per deciliter] refers to the amount of a substance in a bit more than 3 ounces of blood). Values higher than that range for either measurement mean that kidney function is declining.

A *blood urea nitrogen (BUN)* test measures the quantity of nitrogen in your blood that comes from the waste product urea. A BUN is performed to see how well your kidneys are functioning. If your kidneys can't remove urea from the blood, your BUN level will rise.

Measuring *creatinine clearance* can determine how much creatinine your kidneys remove from your body as well as how well your kidneys are functioning. Creatinine clearance is a more precise measure of kidney function than relying on blood measurements alone. To perform a creatinine clearance test, your doctor will ask you to collect your urine over a twenty-four-hour period in a large container. A laboratory will then analyze your urine for creatinine. In addition to a urinalysis, a small amount of your blood will be analyzed for *creatinine*. Your calculated creatinine clearance is expressed as the volume of blood your kidneys completely clear of creatinine per minute. A normal creatinine clearance ranges from 90 to 130 ml/minute. As kidney function declines, creatinine clearance also drops.

Glomerular filtration rate (GFR), the preferred method for assessing kidney function, is a test similar to creatinine clearance. Your doctor or a laboratory can estimate GFR from blood creatinine—taking into account age, gender, race, and body mass—using the GFR calculator provided by the National Kidney Foundation (http://www .kidney.org/professionals/kdoqi/gfr_calculator.cfm; or go to www .kidney.org and link to the calculator from there). Like creatinine clearance, GFR provides more accurate information about kidney function than blood creatinine alone does. Normal values are 80 to 120 ml/minute/1.73m². From the value obtained, your doctor can determine the stage of your kidney disease and can easily monitor its progression without having to obtain a twenty-four-hour urine collection from you each time your blood creatinine is measured. In addition, she can use this information to plan your treatment.

Once kidney failure has been revealed through one of the tests described above, your doctor may refer you to a nephrologist. The National Kidney Foundation's guidelines suggest that patients be referred to a nephrologist when their GFR is less than 30. Your doctor may also refer you to a nephrologist if he is not able to perform all the appropriate diagnostic, treatment, and management recommendations for kidney failure.

If you are happy with your doctor, then her recommended nephrologist will probably be someone you come to trust as well. But personal interactions are subjective, and different patients may view the same doctor differently, for all kinds of reasons. If you sense that you are not getting the nephrologist's full attention, or if the nephrologist will not explain terms, concepts, or the medical care being recommended, or if you feel that your condition is not being properly managed, you may want to consider getting a second opinion from another nephrologist. It may be that you will want to switch doctors, or the second opinion may reinforce your confidence in your current nephrologist.

Table 4.2 displays the stages of kidney disease and outlines a general action plan that your doctor may use for each stage. Stage 1 is defined as the stage when GFR is 90 or higher but there are markers of kidney damage, like protein in the urine or kidney cysts in people who have PKD. Your nephrologist will check your heart's health and will look for any other cardiovascular issues. At Stage 1 your nephrologist will concentrate on finding the cause of your kidney failure and on treating any underlying disease, like diabetes.

Stage 2 is classified by a GFR of 60 to 89. In addition to giving you a diagnosis of your stage, and treating you, your nephrologist will try to slow the decline of your kidney function, perhaps prescribing medications to control your blood pressure or to help treat other underlying diseases. *During Stages 1 and 2, you must follow your doctor's recommendations, even if you don't feel sick.* By doing so, you have the greatest chance of postponing the complete loss of kidney function, perhaps indefinitely. In addition, you may have no symptoms of kidney disease and you may feel well enough to live a normal life.

At Stage 3, with a GFR of 30 to 59, there are more evident complications of chronic kidney disease. For example, you may become anemic, show evidence of bone disease, or have a poor nutritional status. Although it may be years before your kidneys completely

Table 4.2
Sample Clinical Action Plan for Chronic Kidney Disease

Stage	Description	GFR (ml/min/1.73m²)	Action*
	At increased risk	≥ 90 (with CKD risk factors)	Screening, CKD risk reduction
1	Kidney damage with normal or ↑ GFR	≥ 90	Diagnosis and treatment, of comorbid conditions, slowing progression, CVD risk reduction
2	Kidney damage with mild ↓ GFR	60–89	Estimating progression
3	Moderate ↓ GFR	30–59	Evaluating and treating complications
4	Severe ↓ GFR	15–29	Preparation for kidney replacement therapy
5	Kidney failure	< 15 (or dialysis)	Replacement (if anemia present)

Source: Adapted from National Kidney Foundation, "K/DOQI Clinical Practice Guidelines for Chronic Kidney Disease: Evaluation, Classification, and Stratification," *American Journal of Kidney Disease* 39 (2002): S1–S266.

Notes: Shaded area identifies persons who have chronic kidney disease (CKD), defined as pathologic abnormalities or markers of kidney damage lasting at least three months, including abnormalities found in blood or urine tests or imaging studies, and a GFR < 60; unshaded area designates individuals who are at increased risk for developing CKD. Abbreviations: GFR, glomerular filtration rate; CKD, chronic kidney disease; CVD, cardiovascular disease.

*Includes actions of preceding stages.

fail, if at all, your nephrologist will discuss with you the treatment options for kidney failure, including dialysis and transplantation.

If you reach Stage 4, with a GFR of 15 to 29, your nephrologist will prepare you for dialysis by explaining the process and will have you evaluated for a kidney transplant (see chapters 6 and 7). He will explain the drawbacks and benefits of these treatments and help you decide which one is best for you and your lifestyle. It's a painful fact that a transplant may not be available for years, if you don't have a donor. Your doctor can help you plan how to integrate these treatments into your life to make them as unobtrusive as possible.

Stage 5, when GFR is less than 15, means that you must have dialysis or transplantation to live.

Serum creatinine levels are a useful gauge of kidney function, but by themselves they are not a reliable indication of disease. Assessing the degree of kidney decline solely from these levels can be very misleading. When followed over time, they may appear to rise rapidly. However, calculating the GFRs for these values can provide a different picture. Changes in serum creatinine from 1 to 2 in the normal range represent much larger percentage changes in GFR than when they rise from 3 to 4. While on the surface it would seem that a change in the higher levels (3 and 4) would cause more concern than an increase from 1 to 2, we have to consider that a 100 percent change (from 1 to 2) is larger than a 33 percent change (from 3 to 4). It could be many years before you will need dialysis or transplantation. Thus, it is not that kidney function has declined faster, it just seems that way because you are only looking at creatinine, not GFR. In other words, your kidney function is not declining as fast as you may fear it is.

Your doctor will also determine whether you are anemic (see chapter 2). Red blood cells, hemoglobin, and hematocrit are all factors in diagnosing anemia. *Hemoglobin* is a protein in red blood cells that carries oxygen from the lungs to the rest of the body. Normal hemoglobin concentrations are between 14.0 g/dl and 18.0 g/dl. *Hematocrit* measures the percentage of blood volume occupied by red blood cells. Normal hematocrit values are 40 to 54 percent for men and 37 to 47 percent for women. Low hemoglobin or hematocrit values may mean you have anemia, a condition that is common in more advanced stages of kidney disease.

Your Nephrologist

Once you have been referred to a nephrologist, he will become your primary care provider, even though your family physician will continue to be involved in your general care. Your nephrologist may be one of several doctors providing your health care, depending on the underlying disease causing your kidney failure. For example, if you have heart disease, a cardiologist may be monitoring your cardiac health; if you have diabetes, an endocrinologist may be managing your blood sugar; if you have lupus, a rheumatologist may be treating inflammation. Ideally, all of your doctors will work together as a team and will communicate closely with you and with one another.

The stage of kidney disease and the cause of kidney disease determine the recommended treatment. Many people do not see a nephrologist until their kidney disease is fairly advanced, because they do not know they have kidney disease until it reaches a later stage. But if you do see a nephrologist at an early stage, he can focus on the underlying cause and possibly intervene to reduce the progression of kidney failure as well as manage any signs and symptoms you may have.

A first visit to the nephrologist will include a thorough examination of your medical records, as well as assessments of your kidney function, urine, or any diagnosed kidney disease. If you have no diagnosed disease, your nephrologist will begin by identifying the primary cause of your declining kidney function. In addition, assuming that the nephrologist has ruled out acute or short-term kidney failure, she will want to know your stage of chronic kidney disease. With a diagnosis, the nephrologist can work to decrease the rate of loss of kidney function, to control your blood pressure, and, depending on the stage of kidney disease, to manage any complications. (Complications typically begin when your GFR is below 60.) Your nephrologist may also recommend magnetic resonance imaging (MRI) of your kidneys to measure their size or to locate cysts or stones. A kidney biopsy may be necessary to make a diagnosis and to help determine the best way to treat you.

Ask your nephrologist any questions you have about your disease. She should help you understand kidney failure and your long-term prognosis. Your nephrologist can also educate you about new treatments and the latest research that may ultimately lead to slowing the progression of kidney disease.

The information your nephrologist shares with you during your first visit depends on the underlying cause of your kidney failure. If you have diabetes and excrete protein in your urine, your nephrologist will advise you to control your blood sugar and blood pressure with diet and medications. If applicable, your nephrologist will recommend that you lose weight, stop smoking, and take measures to lower your cholesterol.

If you have PKD, you may be newly diagnosed and in the early stages of the disease, with only a few cysts in your kidneys. It could be many years before there is a need for dialysis or a transplant. Moreover, if you are newly diagnosed and in your fifties, you may never need dialysis or transplantation, especially if you have only a few cysts. The discussion of dialysis and transplantation varies greatly, depending on many factors.

By Stage 3, however, you may have lost half of your kidney function. At Stage 3, your nephrologist will probably advise you that you will need dialysis or a transplant in the future.

It is important that you understand the difference between *stability* of kidney function and *level* of kidney function. For example, your nephrologist may be satisfied if your creatinine remains at 3.0. However, he might not always remind you that you have lost more than half of your kidney function, and that being stable with poor kidney function is not normal. GFR almost never improves.

Remember, your nephrologist wants to be reassuring at the same time that he wants you to take care of you. If it has been a while since you discussed your prognosis with your nephrologist, ask him to discuss your future with you.

Managing the Consequences of Kidney Failure

As you read earlier in this chapter, you may encounter a number of consequences involving other organs and processes in your body as your kidney function declines. Although these problems can be worrisome, your nephrologist can help you manage them.

Kidney disease is a primary risk factor for heart disease—including heart attacks—just like smoking and high cholesterol are. As a result, your nephrologist will encourage you to manage your blood pressure and to live a healthy lifestyle. Living a healthy lifestyle is one aspect of your care over which you have total control. You can manage your diet more than almost any other aspect of your life. As your kidneys lose their ability to work properly, eating a heart-healthy diet is essential—along with managing your blood pressure and lowering your cholesterol. If you are obese, lose weight and begin an exercise program. If you smoke tobacco, stop smoking. Get help with weight loss and smoking cessation if you need to.

Depending on the stage of kidney disease, your nephrologist may recommend that you eat a low-salt diet, especially if you have high blood pressure. Failing kidneys cannot eliminate the excess salt intake, and so the soft tissues of the body begin to accumulate fluid. This accumulated fluid, called *edema,* can be uncomfortable, especially if it collects in the legs and ankles. Fluid accumulating in the lungs restricts the airway and can impair breathing. Prescription diuretics can help control your edema as long as you can still pass adequate amounts of urine. Occasionally excessive fluid in the lungs is a medical emergency, requiring hospitalization for removal. Tell your doctor immediately if you have any trouble breathing.

Your nephrologist will recommend a modest restriction of protein in your diet, because a lower-protein diet may slow the progression of kidney disease, especially if you have protein in your urine. You should eat a heart-healthy, high-fiber, low-fat, low-cholesterol diet. You can find more information about diet in chapter 5.

As we learned in chapter 2, kidneys do more than just filter waste products out of the blood. Kidneys also control blood pressure, regulate red blood cell production, maintain the proper acidity in the blood, control potassium and phosphate levels, and activate vitamin D to help build and maintain strong bones. When kidney function deteriorates, complications with the functions described above (and described in more detail below) may arise and may require medical treatment.

Anemia

Low levels of red blood cells, or anemia, is one of the complications of chronic kidney disease. As kidney function declines, the amount of the hormone erythropoietin available to regulate red blood cell production decreases, leading to anemia. People with anemia feel tired, even with adequate sleep. Synthetic, injectable hormone treatments like Epogen, Procrit, or Aranesp (Darbepoetin) may help treat anemia. A health care provider can inject the medication for you or teach you how to do it yourself.

Prescription hormone treatment for anemia is most effective for people with hematocrit ranges from 30 to 33. If your hematocrit is much higher than these levels, hormone treatment may be unsafe, potentially causing heart problems and blood clots. Your nephrologist will carefully monitor your hematocrit to determine whether hormone treatment is right for you.

Blood Acidity

When kidneys can no longer regulate blood acidity, acid builds up, causing acidosis. If you have acidosis, your nephrologist will prescribe sodium bicarbonate (baking soda), which neutralizes the excess acid. You can use either regular baking soda that you find in the grocery store, sodium bicarbonate tablets, or sodium citrate liquid, which the body converts into bicarbonate.

High Potassium and Phosphate

Potassium and phosphate levels in the blood may rise with progressing kidney disease. High potassium and phosphate levels typically occur at Stages 4 and 5. Normal kidneys regulate the amount of *potassium* in the blood by excreting excess amounts. As kidney function declines, however, the kidneys may lose this ability and blood potassium can increase, sometimes to dangerous levels. If high enough, potassium can cause a heart attack. Although you can help lower potassium levels by managing your diet, in some cases, your doctor may prescribe sodium polystyrene sulfonate (Kayexalate) or a diuretic like furosemide (Lasix) to treat excess potassium. A dietitian can help you choose the right kinds of foods to avoid high potassium levels. Your nephrologist will recommend a consultation with a dietician if needed. Most dialysis centers have dieticians available.

Phosphorus in the form of phosphate is important in the production of energy from consumed food. However, the body does not use all of the phosphate ingested and must remove the excess amounts. Normally, the kidneys do that job. As kidney function deteriorates, the kidney cannot eliminate the excess phosphate, so it accumulates and lowers calcium in the blood. In people on or nearing the start of dialysis (see chapters 2 and 6), these deposits can, in the extreme, remove calcium from the bones and lead to osteoporosis. People with high phosphorus may also experience itching. People with high phosphorus levels must reduce phosphate intake (see chapter 6) and may need to take medications to bind ingested phosphate before it can be absorbed. Over-the-counter calcium carbonate tablets like Tums or prescribed drugs like calcium acetate (Phos-Lo) and sevelamer (Renagel) can help control high phosphorus levels.

Low Vitamin D

As you lose kidney function, your body may not make enough kidney-activated vitamin D to maintain sufficient calcium levels to keep your bones strong. In addition, *parathyroid hormone* levels can rise, leaching calcium out of your bones. In reverse to what happens with *excess* phosphate in the blood, *inadequate* levels of calcium can make your bones brittle, causing them to break more easily or begin to hurt. Your nephrologist can treat vitamin D deficiency with several drugs, like paricalcitol (Zemplar) or calcitriol (Rocaltrol), synthetic forms that bypass the need for your kidneys to activate inactive forms of vitamin D (see chapter 2).

The Signs and Symptoms of Failing Kidneys

When our kidneys are working normally, we may be unaware of their great ability to cleanse our bodies of the toxins that accumulate after we digest our food. Urination is the only overt sign that our kidneys work at all. And when our kidneys slowly begin to fail, we can detect, at first, only subtle changes in how we feel. Here are a few of my experiences with kidney failure and a description of how my nephrologist helped me.

During the first three stages of kidney disease, I felt fine. The only health issue I faced during that period was high blood pressure and a kidney infection. My first symptom of kidney failure was fatigue. My fatigue occurred slowly, so initially I did not notice anything unusual. I just assumed I was working too hard or was not getting enough sleep. In time, fatigue became noticeable. By this point I had reached Stage 4 kidney failure.

During the two or three years before I began dialysis, I was so tired that I had difficulty getting up for work every morning, no matter how much sleep I got. Finally, after telling my nephrologist about my fatigue, tests showed that I had become very anemic. With fewer red blood cells carrying oxygen throughout my body, my muscles could no longer do what they needed to do for very long without my feeling debilitated.

My red blood cell count was very low, because I had lost so much of my own erythropoietin (EPO). As a result, my nephrologist prescribed an injectable form of the hormone to produce more red blood cells. Injecting it into my own body was similar to what people with diabetes do—injecting themselves with insulin to normalize their blood sugar. With practice, I found it easy to inject myself with EPO. Besides, I had to do it only once a week, rather than the twice-a-day injections of insulin. After several weeks of injections, I started feeling normal again. In the end, the fatigue I experienced confirmed what my increasing creatinine levels were already telling me: my kidneys were failing and dialysis or transplantation was inevitable.

A year later, my fatigue returned and I began to feel increasingly nauseated and was vomiting frequently. By then, I was approaching Stage 5. Nausea and vomiting were the worst symptoms that I had. To help, my doctor prescribed ondansetron (Zofran), which is used to treat nausea and vomiting in people with cancer who are receiving chemotherapy or radiation treatments. Even this heavy-duty drug could not completely treat my symptoms. I had to tough it out until I could start dialysis or receive a transplant.

In addition to nausea and vomiting, I needed more EPO to keep my anemia under control. Moreover, I required additional medication to control my blood pressure. All of this attention to treatment combined with symptoms sapped my energy, making it difficult for me to do anything. As my kidney failure accelerated, I had to decide, with the help of my nephrologist, when I would start dialysis, because I did not have a kidney donor.

The decision whether to start dialysis or to receive a kidney transplant, if a donor kidney is available, is both a medical and a personal decision. Medically, people usually cannot start dialysis until their GFR is below 15. Medicare will not pay for dialysis or transplantation until GFR is 15 or less, except when your doctor has documented other reasons, like fluid overload, high potassium, or acidosis that cannot be corrected with fluid restriction or medications.

For me, the decision to start dialysis depended mostly on how badly I felt and on knowing that dialysis would require a significant change in my lifestyle. I talked to some people who thought they had waited too long. Although it can take some time, many people feel better after starting dialysis. The decision to get a transplant is usually an easy one, unless you are not medically fit for one. When my kidneys failed, I really had no choice. I had to do something if I wanted to continue living. When I finally faced that decision, I started dialysis. As it turned out, it was not the end of the world. It saved my life.

I do not tell my story to scare you but to make the point that there are many ways to minimize the consequences of kidney disease. You should learn how to prevent or slow the progression of your declining kidney function. This knowledge can extend your healthy time before you have to make life-altering decisions about dialysis or transplantation. Chapter 5 explores the various ways you can change your behavior and various treatments to keep your kidneys working as long as possible.

5

PREVENTING AND POSTPONING KIDNEY FAILURE

Benjamin Franklin wrote that an "ounce of prevention is worth a pound of cure." This adage is certainly true with kidney failure. In chapter 3 we learned that the major causes of kidney failure—diabetes and hypertension—can be prevented. Even an inherited disease like polycystic kidney disease (PKD) has environmental and lifestyle components, where interventions can sometimes extend kidney function, indefinitely in some cases. Who would not want to prevent their kidneys from failing? Certainly, few of us would intentionally live our lives in a way that might cause kidney failure. Many otherwise rational people, however, find it hard to do what is best for their health rather than what they are used to doing—or what they would prefer to do. Beyond human nature, there are several other factors that might circumvent early interventions that might prevent or delay kidney failure.

One of them is not knowing that you are sick. When we are young and healthy, it's easy to neglect our health. Most young people have no medical problems they know about, even though they may be vaguely aware of some that may lurk in the background. That was true for me in my late twenties. After I earned my doctorate, I pursued a research career as a visiting fellow at the National Institutes of Health. My fellowship did not provide health insurance, and I could not afford to buy it. Because I was healthy at the time and did not know I had PKD, I took the chance of doing without health insurance for my two-year fellowship. As a young man I thought I was invincible—that is, until I developed hypertension in my thirties. Even then, I took prescribed medications and went on with my life.

Even when the warning signs of impending disease appear, it can still be difficult to believe that we may eventually face a serious health condition like kidney failure. Denial may prevent us from taking immediate action for our medical condition, especially if we assume that the condition is not serious or that we have plenty of time to address it (see chapter 1). Most people would prefer to focus their attention on more immediate issues. Often it takes a medical crisis to wake us up.

If we accept that we are at risk of a serious medical problem, shouldn't we want to confront it? Not necessarily, because confronting medical conditions is difficult. Nevertheless, the first step in preventing more serious complications down the road is to reach the stage where we accept that *acting now* could save our lives.

We understand enough about the risk factors for kidney failure that we know some things we can do to significantly reduce the chances of kidney failure *before it occurs*. Being educated about health risks is a good start (see chapter 3). In this chapter I outline some specific ways to address these risks. Sound medical practices may reduce the risk of kidney failure and address many other health issues, like the harmful consequences of diabetes, hypertension, and heart disease. In addition to safeguarding your health on your own, you and everyone else need to have regular medical checkups and treatment for any underlying causes of kidney failure.

Weight Loss, Diet, and Exercise

Hypertension is one of the main contributors to kidney failure, no matter what the primary cause of kidney decline. Although factors related to diabetes, glomerular diseases, and PKD can destroy kidney function, hypertension can accelerate the decline. A major contributor to hypertension is obesity.

Obesity can increase blood pressure in several ways. For one, the heart must work harder to move blood through a large body. In addition, the renin-angiotensin and adrenaline systems become overactive (see chapter 2). In people with diabetes, insulin resistance is a factor. Fat deposits can apply pressure on the outside walls of blood vessels, increasing resistance to blood flow. Finally, increased salt consumption accompanies overeating; excess salt intake promotes water retention, further contributing to hypertension. The bottom line? Overweight people at risk of kidney failure must lose weight.

Granted, losing weight is easier said than done. Books and magazines tout various ways to shed unwanted pounds, and I am not going to evaluate their claims. I will confirm the mantra of every weight-reducing diet, however: *to lose weight, you must burn more calories than you consume.* This means adopting a healthy, low-calorie, low-fat diet and an exercise program.

I was once obese. In my early forties, I became too fond of junk food. Over time, I gained 60 to 70 pounds above my ideal weight. I had a poor self-image, but what got my attention was an incident one evening as I climbed a flight of stairs to bed. I felt so winded that I could barely breathe. I realized then that if I did not do something about my weight, I might not make it to my sixties.

In consultation with my physician, I changed my diet and started exercising. Changing my diet took time. My body had become accustomed to all the sugar and fat that I had been eating. Eventually my new diet stuck, and I reached a point where eating junk food made me sick. Sticking to my diet didn't mean I had to deprive myself of anything. When I had a craving for a certain food, I would let myself eat it, but only very small portions. Allowing myself this luxury helped me avoid consuming extra calories.

Beginning an exercise regimen was also a challenge, largely because I did not know how to do it effectively. So I hired a personal trainer who accepted no excuses from me about not coming to the gym as scheduled. The first few months were very frustrating. I did not lose any weight at all for three months, even though I ate a low-calorie diet and vigorously exercised. It took that long to trick my body into accepting my lower caloric intake instead of my usual high caloric consumption. After that, I lost 30 pounds in a few months. Eventually, I lost the extra pounds and returned to a normal weight.

I know firsthand how difficult it is to lose weight. There are no quick tricks, either. To lose weight and keep it off requires a permanent change in lifestyle, involving diet and exercise. You must make losing weight a priority and you must be motivated, disciplined, and determined to get to a healthy weight. With the help of your doctor, a nutritionist, perhaps a personal trainer, and the support of friends and family, you, too, can lose weight. It takes a long-term commitment and patience.

Salt, Protein, and Phosphorus Restriction

Reducing your intake of specific foods may help you lose weight and may also reduce the strain on your kidneys and prolong their function.

The first dietary change that people with kidney disease should make is to restrict salt intake. Most nutritionists recommend that you ingest no more than 2,000 to 2,400 mg of salt each day from all sources. But so much of what we buy and eat is loaded with salt that salt can be difficult to avoid. Eating less salt can be hard to get used to. Like eating fewer calories, you can condition yourself to prefer the taste of foods with less salt. The biggest culprits providing excess salt are meals in restaurants and prepared foods.

Restaurants often serve extremely large portions of food. Restaurant meals are also often excessively salty. While you shouldn't avoid eating in restaurants, there are ways you can minimize your caloric and salt intake. First, if your meal is too large, divide it in half or in thirds and take the rest home for subsequent meals. Avoid ordering menu items that come with sauces, which are often full of fat and salt. You may also ask the chef to avoid salting your food as much as possible. (You can always add some salt to taste if the food is too bland.) Eat grilled or broiled food instead of fried food, which is generally high in fat. (If the grilled or broiled food is coated with fat and salt, however, it may still be unhealthy.) Finally, experiment with healthy cuisines that you may not normally eat. You may discover foods that you really like and that are more nutritious and less salty than your normal fare.

Prepared foods often have too much salt. This is especially true of frozen meals and canned foods and soups. You don't need to avoid these convenience foods completely, but learn how to read the nutrition labels. If you normally eat three meals a day, remember that a single meal cannot contain more than 670 mg of salt and still remain within the daily guideline. Of course, if you eat more than three meals a day—a practice that is often recommended in dieting—each small meal must have proportionally less salt. Several companies, like Healthy Choice and Lean Cuisine, sell frozen meals with lower salt content than other companies' products. Read and compare labels. Canned foods often have a lot of salt, but you can significantly reduce the salt count by discarding any liquid in the cans and by rinsing the contents. Obviously, this approach will not work with canned soups, which generally should be avoided. If you like soup, make your own with fresh ingredients and as little salt as possible.

Reducing protein in the diet may also be helpful in postponing kidney failure, as suggested by considerable evidence obtained from animal studies. Because kidneys normally filter protein and return it to the blood, with lower levels of protein, they do not need to work as hard. People with diabetes or glomerular diseases (where protein spills into the urine, reflecting kidney damage) can improve their health by eating less protein. In addition, you might eat soy or other plant protein, like legumes and whole grains, rather than animal protein. Although researchers have not extensively studied protein intake levels in humans, reducing the amount of protein you consume has little downside risk and might be beneficial to your health. People with advanced kidney failure should exercise caution, however. Reducing your protein intake may result in insufficient caloric intake and may put you at significant risk of malnutrition. Talk to your nephrologist and your dietitian to strike the right balance.

As we learned in chapter 2, phosphorus in the form of phosphate is an important element in many energy-producing reactions of the body. Because we consume more phosphorus than we need, the kidney must excrete the excess amount. Limiting phosphorus intake can help take the load off your kidneys. When a person's kidney function is poor or the person is on dialysis (see chapter 6), it is even more important to limit phosphorus consumption. Cola drinks and dairy products are a main source of phosphorus and may have to be consumed in small amounts only. Rice milk is a suitable substitute for skim milk. Soy milk contains too much phosphorus.

Reading Food Labels

It's easy to eat the wrong foods, in part because we do not understand what's in the food we're eating. Learn to read a food label as one way to help avoid eating harmful foods. Figure 5.1 shows an example of a typical food label—for packaged macaroni and cheese. Several items on the label are particularly pertinent for people with failing kidneys as well as for people trying to lose weight.

First, check the serving size. It can be easy to buy an item that looks as if it is a single serving when it is not. A small package of snacks or bottle of soda represents more than one serving. As figure 5.1 shows, eating the entire item means consuming two servings and double the calories, fat, and salt of the single serving as gauged by the food manufacturer.

If you are limiting fat intake, check the number of calories contributed by fat, which is listed next to the number of total calories per serving. Consider that the label indicates that a single serving contains 110 calories from fat, while there are 250 total calories in the single serving. This means that almost 50 percent of the calories in a single serving comes from fat! And the percentage is often much higher for cheeses and cooking oils, so people who consume a lot of these foods are taking in more fat and calories than they might realize. Check the labels. Look for food where the majority of the calories come from a source other than fat.

Sample Label for Macaroni and Cheese

Start Here

Nutrition Facts
Serving Size 1 cup (228g)
Servings Per Container 2

Amount Per Serving

Calories 250   Calories from Fat 110

% Daily Value*

Limit These Nutrients

	% Daily Value*
Total Fat 12g	18%
Saturated Fat 3g	15%
Trans Fat 1.5g	
Cholesterol 30mg	10%
Sodium 470mg	20%
Total Carbohydrate 31g	10%
Dietary Fiber 0g	0%
Sugars 5g	
Protein 5g	

Get Enough of These Nutrients

Vitamin A	4%
Vitamin C	2%
Calcium	20%
Iron	4%

Quick Guide to % Daily Value

(5% or less is low 20% or more is high)

*Percent Daily Values are based on a 2,000 calorie diet. Your Daily Values may be higher or lower depending on your calorie needs:

Footnote

	Calories:	2,000	2,500
Total Fat	Less than	65g	80g
Sat Fat	Less than	20g	25g
Cholesterol	Less than	300mg	300mg
Sodium	Less than	2,400mg	2,400mg
Total Carbohydrate		300g	375g
Dietary Fiber		25g	30g

Figure 5.1. A Typical Food Label

Fat, cholesterol, and sodium—the substances labeled "Limit These Nutrients" in figure 5.1—should be consumed only in small amounts if you have kidney disease. A high-fat and high-salt diet can lead to the formation of fat deposits in blood vessels and to high blood pressure, heart disease, and some cancers. Some fats, however—those designated as monounsaturated or polyunsaturated, like olive oil—may be beneficial. The nutrients labeled "Get Enough" are healthy and should be consumed in large amounts. Some people do not get enough vitamins and minerals in their diets and may need to take supplements to satisfy their daily requirements.

The footnote at the bottom of a food label provides basic nutritional information, based on the advice of experts, on the upper and lower limits you should consume daily, depending on the number of calories consumed. Values for fat, cholesterol, and sodium represent the upper limit, whereas the dietary value for fiber is the minimum daily amount most people need. Based on those guidelines, the percentage of the daily values provided by the food (in this case, the packaged macaroni and cheese) is listed by each item. A value of 5 percent or less is low, whereas 20 percent or more is high. These values provide comparisons among food items so it's easier to identify which foods are best for your diet.

Unfortunately, food manufacturers are not required to list the potassium or phosphorus content per serving on their food labels. This poses a unique challenge for people with kidney disease. Some manufacturers list them voluntarily, helping you to know which products are safe to eat and which items are to be avoided. Chapter 6 lists some foods that are high and low in potassium and phosphorus.

Managing Your Blood Pressure

Although obesity can contribute to hypertension, not everyone with hypertension is overweight. In obese people and in people with hypertension, however, diet alone may not lower blood pressure to the desirable 120/80 or below. Some people must take medications to control high blood pressure.

Recent research suggests that maintaining a blood pressure of 125/75 can postpone kidney failure for years. Luckily, the treatment of hypertension has evolved over the last four decades, and today there are many classes of medications working through different mechanisms to control blood pressure. Although a single medication may be effective in controlling hypertension, clinical research has shown that a combination of medications may be needed to reduce high blood pressure. Working through different mechanisms, some classes of medications may be better than others in protecting kidney function.

In chapter 2, I discussed a biochemical process initially mediated by the kidney that can cause hypertension. This process involves the release of the hormone renin from the kidney. Renin activates angiotensin synthetic pathways, whereby angiotensin II constricts blood vessels and increases blood pressure.

There are two ways to interfere with the ability of angiotensin II to elevate blood pressure: block the production of angiotensin II or reduce the actions of angiotensin II on blood vessels. Medications that block the formation of angiotensin II are called *angiotensin-converting enzyme, or ACE, inhibitors*. One such medication is lisinopril (Zestril and Prinivil). These drugs have been in use for many years, have been well studied, and might be especially beneficial in protecting kidney function. Another drug that blocks angiotensin II receptors is losartan (Cozaar). This drug also reduces blood pressure effectively. Because one of these drug classes may not be sufficient to lower blood pressure to the desired level, the effectiveness of combining both classes of drugs is currently under investigation for treating PKD.

The other drug classes that can reduce blood pressure do so directly by relaxing blood vessels or altering heart rate and the amount of blood the heart ejects with each beat (cardiac output)—or through a combination of these effects. At the cellular level, all of these drugs work by blocking receptors that normally translate the signals of the body's hormones or chemical transmitters into a physiological response. Two classes of drugs that lower blood pressure act on the heart and, to some extent, on the blood vessels directly. One class, named beta-blockers, slows the heart rate and reduces cardiac output, thereby lessening the burden on the heart and reducing blood pressure. Atenolol (Tenormin) is a commonly prescribed beta-blocker. The other class of drugs acting on the heart and blood vessels includes the calcium-channel blockers. These drugs prevent the inflow of calcium into cells that stimulate the contraction of muscle in the heart and blood vessels, thereby lowering blood pressure.

As we learned earlier, hypertension is often difficult to treat with only one class of drug. To control your hypertension, you may need to take several different classes of drugs with different actions, and possibly others as well, including, for example, diuretics (water pills) like hydrochlorothiazide (Microzide); alpha-blockers like terazosin (Hytrin), which acts directly on the blood vessels, or others, which work through the brain; and minoxidil (Loniten), which directly opens blood vessels. Your doctor may determine the best treatment for your hypertension by trial and error.

Experimental Medications and Clinical Trials

Preventing kidney failure depends on effectively treating the underlying causes of kidney failure. There are many ways to treat hypertension in a person who has no other underlying diseases. However, there are not as many ways to treat diabetes, glomerular diseases, and PKD. Clinical researchers are always working to develop new, more effective drugs. They do this by first studying relevant mechanisms in animal trials. If the results are promising, they move ahead to clinical trials using human volunteers. The federal government has established a website that lists current clinical trials: www. clinicaltrials.gov. On this website you can find information about current research and applications. There are some promising new approaches to treating the underlying diseases that can lead to kidney failure. Here are a few examples of what clinical researchers are pursuing. (When reading these descriptions, keep in mind that, in scientific and medical research, new treatment possibilities emerge while others become dead ends.)

Diabetes

The first line of treatment for diabetes is controlling glucose and insulin levels. For people with mild diabetes, a healthy diet is the first step. The body's supply of glucose and insulin is further regulated through medications that are taken orally. People with Type 1 diabetes take insulin either intramuscularly (as an injection into muscle tissue) or subcutaneously (by using an infusion pump under the skin that continuously releases insulin). None of these treatments is a cure for diabetes; clinical trials are under way to find better treatments or a cure for both Type 1 and Type 2 diabetes.

Researchers are working to develop better drugs that can control cellular responsiveness to insulin. People with Type 2 diabetes are insulin resistant and may benefit from oral medications that improve insulin responsiveness. Insulin responsiveness is a prime target for research. Although these types of drugs have been available for decades, they have not been very effective in people with severe diabetes. For these people, insulin injections are needed to control blood glucose levels. Future drugs may be more effective in controlling insulin resistance, meaning that more people with diabetes can eliminate or postpone the need to take insulin. In the long term, these drugs may reduce the number of people with diabetes experiencing kidney failure.

Clinical studies on Type 1 diabetes are looking for better treatment options to protect the insulin-producing beta cells from being destroyed by the body's own antibodies. The current treatment approach of suppressing the immune system, which interferes with all immune reactions, makes people more vulnerable to infections. The goal of the latest research is to find specific pathways in the immune response that attack beta cells rather than the immune system as a whole. Research is slowly identifying the pathways to the best targets for therapeutic intervention as well as effective new medications.

Another way to treat Type I diabetes is to desensitize the specific immune response that damages beta cells, so that the pathway is less responsive to autoimmune attack. Desensitizing the immune response also reduces the chance that a transplanted organ will be rejected by the body. I participated in such a clinical trial when I received my kidney transplant (see chapter 7). In islet transplants, pancreatic islet cells from deceased donors are infused into a patient to restore insulin secretion without the patient needing to use steroids to suppress system-wide immune responses.

Glomerular Diseases

New treatments for glomerular diseases are emerging, too. The approach of these treatments varies depending on the original source of the disease (see chapter 3). Glomerular diseases are inflammatory diseases that lead to scarring of the glomerulus, and most of the treatment options reduce this inflammation using steroids. Most clinical trials on inflammation focus on inflammatory diseases like lupus. Here, similar to the studies of Type I diabetes, researchers are examining pathways within the immune system to find the most selective approach to minimize or slow the scarring, without using steroids.

One clinical trial is testing a drug that reduces scar formation. Unlike drugs that suppress the immune system, this drug (pirfenidone) acts by blocking the development of scar tissue. The goal is to prevent further scarring in people with declining kidney function.

Polycystic Kidney Disease

Clinical trials to find medications to retard cyst growth in PKD patients are pursuing what is perhaps the most promising approach for treating a major cause of kidney failure. Having developed a better understanding of the underlying mechanisms of how cysts form in the kidneys, researchers have been looking for ways to shrink the size of the cysts. In addition to a multi-center trial combining drugs that act on the angiotensin system, as discussed earlier, other studies are taking additional approaches.

The most advanced of these clinical trials involves blocking the action of the hormone *vasopressin*. Vasopressin, which is released from the pituitary gland to conserve fluid in the body, does so by stimulating cellular mechanisms that can cause cyst formation and growth in people with mutations in their PKD genes (see chapter 3). Indeed, vasopressin levels are higher in PKD patients. An inhibitor of vasopressin can retard cyst formation in a mouse model of PKD. Tolvaptan, an inhibitor of vasopressin, is currently in Phase III clinical trials to determine how effective and safe it is in treating PKD.

Other drugs are being developed to inhibit the size and number of cysts by blocking their blood supply, without which they die. A similar strategy has been successful for treating some types of cancer. One study uses a drug called sirolimus to suppress the immune system in people receiving organ transplants. Researchers found that PKD kidneys and livers shrank after transplant in patients taking sirolimus, unlike what happens when such patients take other immunosuppressants. If this drug works in blocking cyst formation and growth in humans, it could help with the development of new drugs without an immunosuppressant effect.

New research on the underlying causes of kidney failure and the development of potential treatments offer hope to people in fear of losing their kidney function and of facing dialysis or transplantation. Someday, we hope, there will be no need for dialysis clinics and transplant lists and less need for expensive and invasive medical interventions. In the future, the lives of many people with kidney diseases will improve.

In the meantime, people approaching kidney failure must examine the choices available to replace their impending kidney failure. Chapters 6 and 7 cover what you can expect with dialysis and transplantation, and introduce some coping skills that I found helpful.

6

DIALYSIS

Until recent decades, few seriously ill people got a second chance at life. It wasn't until the twentieth century that effective treatments were developed for many diseases. Now, antibiotics and other medical interventions routinely preserve life for many who might otherwise die. Like people with serious infections and people with cancer, people with kidney failure are now having much longer life expectancies than they would have had in the past. In the past, the kidneys of people with kidney failure deteriorated to the point where *uremia*, an excessive buildup of toxins in the blood, resulted in death.

Today, however, there are treatments for kidney failure, including dialysis. Although tested as early as the nineteenth century, dialyzing blood to reduce uremia only became a useful treatment for chronic kidney failure in the 1960s. Now dialysis is in use all over the United States and is available to anyone who needs it. According to the latest statistics from the National Institutes of Health, more than 381,000 people were on some form of dialysis at the end of 2008.[1]

There are two forms of dialysis to treat kidney failure: peritoneal dialysis and hemodialysis. Both forms of dialysis move toxins
across a barrier through which only some substances can pass. The
following section explains the basic concepts of dialysis.

How Dialysis Works

Dialysis involves filtration. Start with a basic concept: imagine a tank
of water into which you carefully place a drop of ink in one cor-
ner of the tank. The concentrated ink tends to diffuse over time
throughout the entire container of water until it reaches the same
concentration in all parts of the tank (figure 6.1, top).

Now insert a barrier, through which nothing can pass, in the
middle of the tank. The ink diffuses throughout only half the container, as shown in figure 6.1 (bottom). If, however, you punch tiny
holes into the barrier, ink will flow through them—as long as the ink
molecules are smaller than the holes. If the molecules are smaller,
they disperse throughout the entire container of water (just like in
figure 6.1, top). If the holes are too small for the ink molecules to
pass through, the ink remains on one side of the barrier (figure 6.1,
bottom).

Increasing the volume of the left side of the tank causes the ink
to diffuse faster through the barrier until the *concentration* of ink is
equal on both sides, while the *amount* of ink is reduced on the right
side (see figure 6.2). For example, if you place 3 grams of ink in the
right side of the tank with 1 liter of water and the ink moves through
the barrier to the other side with 2 liters of water, the concentration
of ink will eventually be equal on both sides of the barrier. This
means only 1 gram remains on the original side of the barrier, and
the remaining 2 grams have crossed the barrier. Thus, on the original side, the concentration of ink declined from $3\,g/l$ to $1\,g/l$, while
on the other side the concentration rose from $0\,g/2\,l$ to $2\,g/2\,l$, or

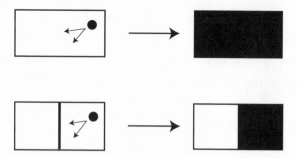

Figure 6.1. Dialysis as Filtration I. With no barriers, a substance will diffuse uniformly (*top*). If a barrier is added, diffusion will only occur in half the container (*bottom*).

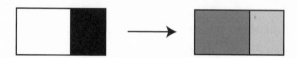

Figure 6.2. Dialysis as Filtration II. This figure shows the *amount* of ink on each side of the barrier rather than the *concentration* of ink. Since the concentration would be equal on each side, if concentrations (rather than amounts) of ink were illustrated, both sides would be the same color, as in the top part of figure 6.1.

1g/l. (Figure 6.2 shows the *amount* of ink on each side of the barrier rather than the *concentration* of ink. Because the concentration would be equal on each side, if concentrations were illustrated, both sides would be the same shade, as in the top part of figure 6.1.)

This concept, called *dialysis*, has been used for years by biochemists to purify chemicals. Similar to the ink analogy, dialysis involves a semi-permeable membrane (a barrier with holes) that allows some substances to pass through and not others, depending on the size of the molecules involved. To accomplish this, the chemical needing purification is placed into a small sac made of the membranous material (the barrier from above) through which the substance to be purified cannot pass. Next, the sac is placed in a volume of appropriate solution much larger than the volume of solution in the sac. The impurities that can pass through the membrane will flow until the concentration is equal on both sides of the membrane, but reducing their amount inside the sac. For maximum efficiency, the solution is changed frequently to allow for the greatest removal of the contaminants in the sac. When successively repeating the exchanges, nearly all of the impurities will eventually be removed.

This is the same basic approach to filtering the blood of people with kidney failure. Early studies in the 1940s, using this principle of dialysis to clean human blood, used pig intestines as the semipermeable membrane, with the blood passing through the interior part. The intestines were placed in big wooden vats of solution composed of salts and buffers compatible with blood. Other laboratories tried using cellophane. The idea was to remove the toxins without removing cells and important proteins from the blood. This approach proved more difficult than simple biochemical dialysis, but over time, with further refinements and miniaturizing the process, the modern forms of dialysis were born.

Today, peritoneal dialysis and hemodialysis are the most common forms of dialysis. Hemodialysis is more routinely used, but increasing numbers of patients are choosing peritoneal dialysis because of its advantages. There are disadvantages to both forms of dialysis, however; these are covered in depth later in this chapter.

Peritoneal Dialysis

The principles of peritoneal dialysis remain the same as described above, but the application is a bit more complicated. Like the biochemical approach to dialysis, *peritoneal dialysis* takes advantage of the semi-permeable membrane that lines the peritoneal cavity of the abdomen. Some substances can pass through it, others cannot.

Tiny blood vessels are embedded in this peritoneal membrane. The blood from the body is analogous to the contents of the membranous sac described above. A solution, called the *dialysate*, is placed in the abdomen, allowing the toxins in the blood to flow through the peritoneal membrane into the solution (see figure 6.3). This occurs because the concentration of toxins in the blood is higher than it is in the dialysate (as in figure 6.2). To avoid loss of needed substances in the blood, the dialysate contains salts and buffers in concentrations equivalent to those normally found in the blood, creating equal concentrations of these substances on both sides of the membrane.

Because fluid balance is compromised in people with kidney failure, dialysis must also remove excess water from the body. In peritoneal dialysis, the dialysate contains glucose (sugar) to help remove the excess water. Because the concentration of glucose exceeds the concentration in the blood and does not appreciably pass into the body, excess fluid in the blood flows through the peritoneal membrane into the dialysate to dilute the glucose. To remove more fluid, higher concentrations of glucose are needed. The rate of diffusion of toxins into the dialysate declines with time, so the dialysate must be exchanged up to five times a day in order to maximize the removal of the toxins.

Before peritoneal dialysis can be performed, a surgeon must place a special *catheter* inside the abdominal wall (see figure 6.4). The part of the catheter that is inside the abdominal wall is either straight or curled like a pig's tail, and has holes in it, whereas on the outside the catheter is straight, solid, and flexible and has a hole only at the outside tip. The hole in the abdomen through which the catheter exits is known as the *exit site*. The subcutaneous and peritoneal cuffs hold the catheter in place, and are sewn into the abdominal wall. With peritoneal dialysis it is crucial to avoid in-

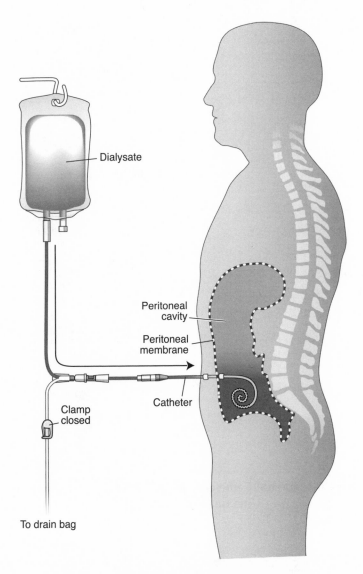

Dialysate

Peritoneal cavity

Peritoneal membrane

Catheter

Clamp closed

To drain bag

Figure 6.3. Dialysate Flowing into the Abdomen

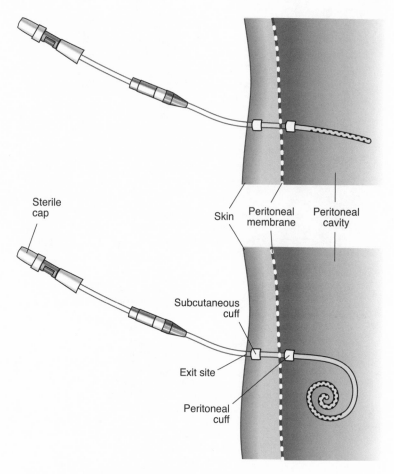

Figure 6.4. Straight Catheter *(top)* **and Curled Catheter** *(bottom)*
Used for Peritoneal Dialysis

fections, which can occur because either the catheter or the exit
site becomes contaminated. After the catheter has been in place
for about two weeks, dialysis can begin. Once an exchange has
been completed, a sterile cap with an antiseptic (like Betadyne) on
the inside is screwed onto the outside end of the catheter (on the
left ends of the catheters in figure 6.4) until the next exchange.

A surgeon has flexibility on where to place the catheter. Unfortunately, I did not talk with my surgeon about placement because I did not know that I could. As a result, when I received a peritoneal catheter, it was placed at my waistline. Wearing pants, with the subcutaneous and peritoneal cuffs directly under my belt, was very uncomfortable. Talk with your surgeon about what options he or she can provide for catheter placement that will minimize discomfort.

Continuous Ambulatory Peritoneal Dialysis (CAPD)

To perform exchanges, you need good manual dexterity, but there are devices to help people with physical limitations. There are even devices that help blind people with exchanges.

Peritoneal dialysis is typically begun using a procedure known as *continuous ambulatory peritoneal dialysis* (CAPD), in which dialysis occurs throughout the day between changes of the dialysis solutions (called *exchanges*). Exchanging solutions is relatively simple—it is a process that takes about twenty minutes, once you are used to it. What follows is the description of a typical procedure for performing exchanges to give you an idea of what is involved.[2] (*Note: The following description is not a substitute for appropriate training by a qualified dialysis health care provider. Talk to your doctor about the best way to perform your exchanges.*) The exchange process must be sterile, so you must make every effort to avoid contamination. Hand washing with antibacterial soap or other suitable decontaminant is required at critical steps in the process. You may also want to dry your hands with a fresh paper towel rather than a cloth towel, to reduce possible contamination from the soiled cloth. Your dialysis center may provide you with an ultraviolet lamp to sterilize the connections between the tubing and your catheter.

Dialysis bags contain sterile solutions and come in sealed outer bags. After washing your hands, you will open the outer bag and

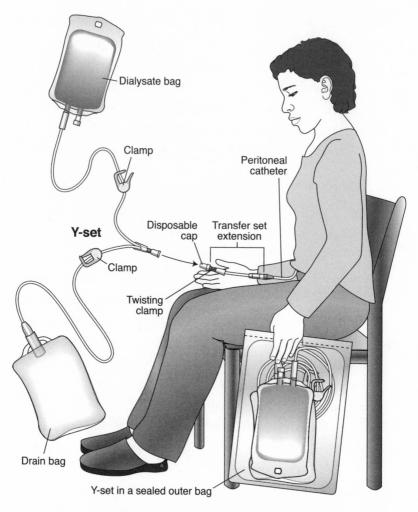

Figure 6.5. Y-Set Used in Dialysis

remove its contents. Bags of dialysis solution include an attached drain bag, collectively known as a Y-set (see figure 6.5). Before starting, warm the dialysis solution to body temperature (easily done in a microwave oven). Warm solution will help prevent abdominal cramping. Attach the fluid-filled bag to a bag pole, and start your exchange.

After washing your hands and drying them with a paper towel, remove and discard the cap on the catheter. Then, attach the catheter to the system, which has a tube to the drain bag and one to the bag containing fresh dialysate. Before flow can occur, break two seals—one on the dialysis bag and one attached to the catheter. After allowing some dialysate to pass through the lines to prime the system (see the upper left side of figure 6.6), clamp the line to the dialysate bag and open the catheter line to allow drainage of your peritoneal fluid (see the upper right side of figure 6.6).

Once drainage is complete, unclamp the line to the dialysate bag to allow flow of some fresh solution into the drain bag to remove bubbles (see the lower left side of figure 6.6), clamp the tube to the drain bag, and then allow flow of fresh dialysate into your abdomen (see the lower right side of figure 6.6). Because the force of gravity helps the dialysate to flow more easily, hang the bag above your head. When the bag is empty, clamp the tube from the dialysate bag and wash your hands again. Then, detach the catheter from the exchange system and immediately screw a fresh cap containing Betadyne on the catheter. Finally, empty the drain bag and then discard the whole system. At this point, your exchange is complete.

Dialysis exchanges can be done almost anywhere you can find privacy. Avoid doing exchanges in public bathrooms or other places where there might be contamination. It is also best not to have people in the same room while you are exchanging—again, because of the risk of contamination.

If you work while on peritoneal dialysis, you will have to find a way to do exchanges in an office or comparable room. If there is a drop ceiling, you can attach the dialysate bags to the ceiling grid with an S-hook, like a plant holder. Otherwise, you may use a bag pole. During exchanges, you can continue working as long as you have privacy. To minimize the number of exchanges at work, do

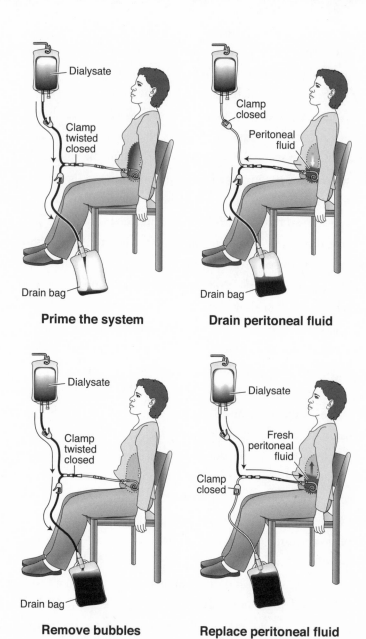

Prime the system

Drain peritoneal fluid

Remove bubbles

Replace peritoneal fluid

Figure 6.6. Dialysis Exchange with Peritoneal Dialysis

the first one as soon as you get up in the morning at home, one just before lunch at the office, one just before leaving for home at the end of the workday or when you first get home, and the last one just before going to bed.

This scenario may not work for everyone. For example, if you do not have your own office or another suitable place to perform exchanges, you may not be a candidate for CAPD. Continuous cyclic peritoneal dialysis may be a better alternative.

Continuous Cyclic Peritoneal Dialysis (CCPD)

Like CAPD, *continuous cyclic peritoneal dialysis (CCPD)* can be a useful option. CCPD uses a machine, called a cycler, which performs exchanges during the night while you are asleep (see figure 6.7). The machine (manufactured by Baxter International, Inc., in Deerfield, Illinois) consists of several parts: (1) a dialysis bag heater; (2) a peristaltic pump inside the machine; (3) a place for a cassette (behind the door in figure 6.8); and (4) a computer (behind the control panel in figure 6.8) to run everything. The cassette controls the flow of fluid from dialysate bags to the abdomen and channels used dialysate to waste. All of the tubing attached to the cassette is needed for dialysis (see the disposable dialysis set in figure 6.9). The cassette works with the peristaltic pump to roll the fluids through the tubing. The computer is programmed to direct the flow either to waste or from one of the dialysis bags.

The rules for use of a cycler are similar to the rules for CAPD, especially when it comes to cleanliness. With practice and training on how the machine works and how to avoid contamination, you can set up the cycler for use in about ten minutes. First, place a 5-liter dialysis bag on top of the cycler where the heater is located. Next, put the cassette in its receptacle and attach the drain line, routing it to a drain, like a toilet, sink, or bathtub. Before attaching

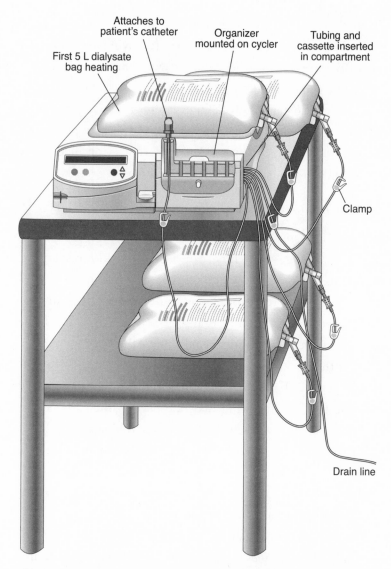

Figure 6.7. Cycler Used in Continuous Cyclic Peritoneal Dialysis

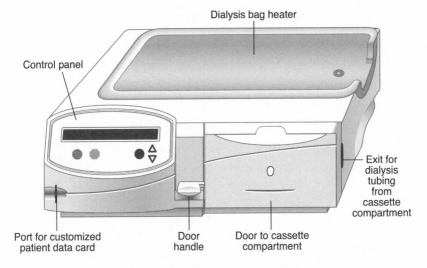

Figure 6.8. Parts of the Cycler

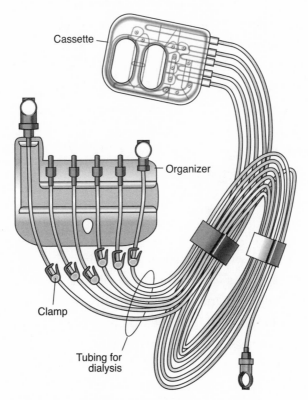

Figure 6.9. Organizer and Tubing of the Cycler

the appropriate tubes to the dialysis bags, wash your hands to avoid contaminating the bags when you insert the tubes. When the cycler has filled the tubing with fluid, wash your hands again, remove and discard the cap on your catheter, and then attach it to the tube at the far left of the organizer (see figure 6.9).

Once the cycler is activated, you can go to sleep. While sleeping, if you turn more than once in succession in the same direction, you might become entangled in the tubing or crimp the tube. If this happens, an alarm will sound to awaken you, and the cycler will stop itself, as a safety measure. Train yourself to roll only back and forth when you want to change your sleeping position.

While you are asleep, the cycler does several exchanges as programmed on the computer, based on your nephrologist's prescription. As the amount of dialysate in the bag on the heater declines, the computer begins pumping dialysate from the other bags, so that the heater can warm the solution from those bags before use. After washing your hands the next morning, detach your catheter from the cycler and screw on a fresh cap containing Betadyne. To complete the process, discard all the plastic tubing and the cassette. This process at first seems complicated but it becomes less so with practice. The biggest advantage of CCPD is that fewer exchanges are needed during the day, especially if you still have some residual kidney function.

Monitoring the Effectiveness of Peritoneal Dialysis

Dialysis is a prescribed treatment and, just like with other prescriptions, its effectiveness needs to be monitored. Nephrologists use two methods to determine how efficiently your treatment removes wastes from your blood. One test is the creatinine and urea clearance. This test is similar to the test your doctor requested to determine your kidney function before your kidneys failed (see chapter 4). To have the test now, you will collect all of the dialysis bags over a twenty-four-hour period as well as any urine you still produce in a large container. When you take the specimens in for analysis, you will be asked to provide a blood sample to determine how much creatinine and urea were removed from your blood.

Another way to measure the efficacy of your dialysis treatment is through a *peritoneal equilibrium test (PET)*. In this test, you will be asked to provide a sample of dialysate at hourly intervals for up to four hours. The dialysate will be tested. The rate at which dialysis removes urea and creatinine from your blood and the extent to which your body absorbs sugar from the dialysate will tell your nephrologist how many exchanges you need to maximize the effectiveness of treatment. From this test your nephrologist can determine if your peritoneal membrane is a rapid transporter or a slow transporter. If it is a rapid transporter, your blood can more easily absorb glucose from the dialysate. This feature can make it difficult to maintain your blood sugar if you have diabetes; as a result, a person with diabetes needs more frequent exchanges. If your membrane is a slow transporter, however, you would benefit from fewer exchanges, with the dialysate remaining in your abdomen for a longer period.

Both CAPD and CCPD offer a great deal of freedom compared to hemodialysis. However, peritoneal dialysis may not be for everyone. Many nephrologists do not offer peritoneal dialysis as an option because some of their patients have developed *peritonitis* (an inflammation of the lining of the abdomen) from it. But peritoneal dialysis is worth considering if you have the discipline to keep up with all of the exchanges and observe the routines necessary to maintain the required cleanliness. Your nephrologist will help you weigh the pros and cons of peritoneal dialysis (including peritonitis, covered later in this chapter) and will help you decide if peritoneal dialysis is right for you.

Hemodialysis

Hemodialysis works on a principle similar to that of peritoneal dialysis, except the blood is cycled outside the body through a special filter, called a *dialyzer*, by a machine that is usually located in a dialysis center (see figure 6.10). Unlike peritoneal dialysis, which is a

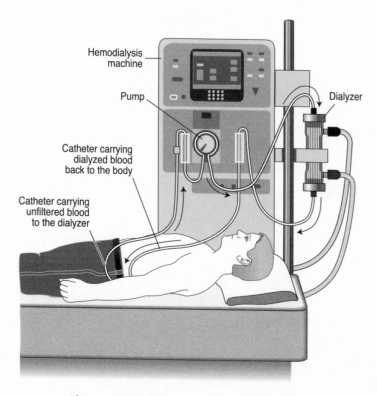

Figure 6.10. Dialyzer Used in Hemodialysis

continuous form of dialysis, hemodialysis is intermittent. Thus, fluid, toxins, and electrolyte imbalances build up between sessions of hemodialysis, which means that the patient must restrict fluid intake and limit some foods. Most patients go to a center three times a week, with each dialysis session typically lasting three to four hours.

Some dialysis centers offer home hemodialysis. If you have someone who can help you set up the machine, insert the needles into your fistula or graft, and monitor your session, home hemodialysis may be an attractive option, especially if you cannot schedule dialysis around work or if your center is not open late in the day. In addition to regular four-hour, three-day-a-week sessions, you may be a candidate for daily dialysis, which would reduce the accumulation of fluid and toxins between sessions. Home hemodialysis sessions last two hours each day, or they can be performed during the night while you sleep. Research suggests that daily hemodialysis may provide a better outcome than three-day-a-week, in-center sessions, since it is a more continuous form of hemodialysis. An increasing number of patients dialyze at home, as long as their dialysis center can provide adequate oversight. To dialyze at home, you must have a person assisting you each time you dialyze, to monitor the treatment in case you experience bleeding or a drop in blood pressure. If your center offers home hemodialysis, consult your nephrologist to see if it is a good choice for you.

The core of hemodialysis is the dialyzer, also known as an artificial kidney. The filter is composed of tiny filaments (semi-permeable membranes) through which the blood passes (see figure 6.11). These filaments are bathed in a continuously flowing dialysate containing salts and buffers in concentrations to avoid excessive loss of these substances from the blood. This process in hemodialysis is analogous to the presence of dialysate in the abdomen when using

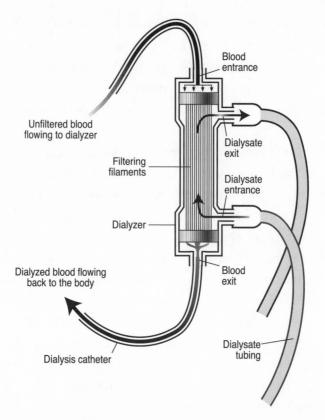

Figure 6.11. Filaments Comprising the Filter of the Dialyzer

peritoneal dialysis. The blood cells and large molecules pass through the dialyzer and return to the body, while the toxins flow freely through the pores in the filaments and wash away.

Vascular Accesses for Dialysis

If you are to receive hemodialysis on a regular basis, your nephrologist or a surgeon must perform a surgical procedure to access your blood supply; blood will be drawn, pumped through the dialysis machine and dialyzer, and then returned to your body. Typically, an access is placed when the estimated GFR is below 30. With suf-

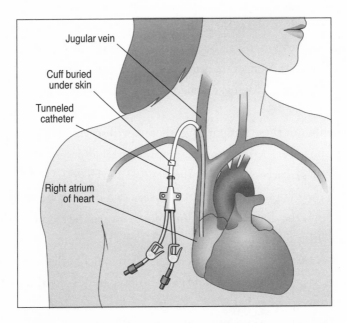

Figure 6.12. Tunneled, Cuffed Hemodialysis Catheter

ficient advance notice, most people can have a permanent access placed (see below). Initially, however, you may need a simple, temporary catheter placed in a large vein in your upper chest or groin. There are two types of dialysis catheter: the untunneled (above the skin) and the tunneled (below the skin) cuffed catheter.

If you need dialysis immediately, you may get an untunneled catheter placed through the right internal jugular vein in your neck into the right atrium of your heart or through the femoral vein in your groin. Your nephrologist, interventional radiologist, or surgeon will perform the procedure while you are under local anesthesia. You may experience a brief, temporary fluttering in your heart if the tip of the catheter contacts heart muscle in the atrium. Untunneled catheters can be used only for a few days to a few weeks, because they tend to come loose, fall out, or become infected.

Tunneled, cuffed catheters may be used for a few weeks to a few months (see figure 6.12). Buried under the skin, the tunneled catheter is larger and longer than an untunneled catheter and is less likely to be dislodged. Moreover, sealed against bacteria, it is less likely to become infected.

Neither of these temporary catheters will serve you for the long term, however. A more permanent and stable access is needed. Two types of access are used: the fistula and the graft. For both of these, the dialysis technician will insert two needles, one to draw blood into the dialysis tubing, and one to return the blood. Both of them will provide a more efficient dialysis treatment than catheters, because the blood can be cleaned more quickly. Planning for a fistula or graft should be done early, to prepare for the time when dialysis will be needed.

To create a *fistula,* a surgeon joins an artery in an arm or groin directly to a vein (see figure 6.13). This procedure is done while you are under anesthesia. Over six to eight weeks, the pressure on the vessel increases, thickening the wall, and then enlarging the vein, making it easier for a dialysis nurse or technician to place the large needles for dialysis. The fistula is the most desirable access to have. Because the fistula is created from your own tissues, it is more resistant to infection, lasts the longest, and has the least number of complications, compared to the other accesses.

The *graft* is a Gore-Tex tube that a surgeon places under the skin, attaching one end of the tube to an artery in your arm or groin and the other end to a vein (see figure 6.14). In this way the procedure is like the fistula procedure, and it, too, is done while you are under anesthesia. The graft may be used sooner than the fistula— generally you can use it after a two-week recovery period. Grafts are not as good as fistulas for dialysis and are more likely to be-

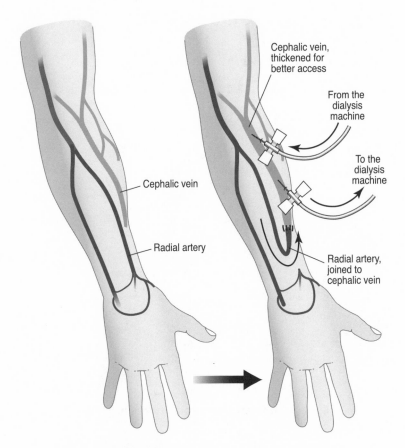

Figure 6.13. Fistula Joining an Artery and a Vein

come infected than fistulas. They are a good substitute if the veins are too small for creating a fistula, however.

Fistulas and grafts use needles with larger internal diameters than catheters, which allows the blood to move faster through the dialyzer. Dialysis is more efficient when blood can pass many times through the dialyzer during a session. However, inserting these larger needles can be painful. To help ease the pain, a dialysis nurse or technician can numb the injection site using a local anesthetic

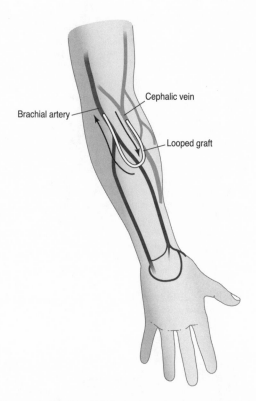

Figure 6.14. Graft Joining an Artery and a Vein

prior to insertion. In order to avoid clotting of the access, the tubing, and the dialyzer, *heparin* (a blood thinner) is injected into the access tubing. As a result, you may experience some bleeding from your access after dialysis. The staff in your center can minimize blood loss by applying pressure to the site using clamps. Some dialysis centers have special bandages containing a substance that helps clot blood.

Monitoring the Effectiveness of Hemodialysis

As with peritoneal dialysis, nephrologists must determine how effective hemodialysis treatments are. Nephrologists use two measures for this purpose: the *urea reduction rate (URR)* and the *Kt/V*.

For the URR, the dialysis technician draws a blood sample from a port on the dialysis machine at the beginning and at the end of dialysis treatment, and sends the blood samples to a lab to determine how much urea is in each sample. The URR is then calculated. A good URR is at least 0.65, which means that the treatment is removing at least 65 percent of urea from the blood.

Kt/V provides the best estimate of the effectiveness of your dialysis treatment. "K" stands for urea clearance during dialysis, "t" for time, and "V" for volume. The calculation of Kt/V is too technical to discuss here. Suffice it to say that, unlike the URR, Kt/V accounts for wide variations in weight among patients by determining the volume of water in the body and the nutritional status. Thus, the Kt/V provides a more accurate measure of effectiveness of a treatment. Good Kt/V values are at least 1.2 to 1.4, but higher values are not more beneficial. Using the Kt/V, a nephrologist can modify a prescription to maximize the efficiency of a dialysis session and help you feel better.

Your nephrologist has several ways to improve the quality of your treatment. For example, he can control the flow rate of your blood through the dialyzer. If you have a fistula or graft, he can increase your flow rate to obtain more dialysis for your time at the center. Another way to improve your treatment is to increase the time on dialysis. Finally, your nephrologist can order a larger dialyzer to allow more purification of blood each time it cycles through.

Monitoring Your Health

Whether using peritoneal dialysis or hemodialysis, your health must be monitored closely. Your nephrologist will assess whether your dialysis prescription is optimal, and she will also help you stay as healthy as possible, so you can feel your best and participate in many of your regular activities. Your laboratory measures provide an open window into your health that will help your nephrologist treat you appropriately.

As we learned before, some of these measures still must be monitored. For example, urea (the BUN number on a lab report) and creatinine levels reveal how well dialysis is cleaning your blood. If these levels are too high, you may need to adjust your diet, or your nephrologist may need to change your medications. Potassium levels are important in regulating heartbeat. If your potassium becomes too high, you could experience an irregular heartbeat or, in extreme cases, a heart block, resulting from a profound slowing of the heart rate. Calcium, phosphorus, and parathyroid hormone levels reflect your bone health. If phosphorous and parathyroid hormone levels are too high, you may have to limit further your phosphorus-rich foods or take higher doses of phosphate binders. Your nephrologist will also monitor your red blood cell count and iron levels. If you become anemic, you may require iron supplementation or erythropoietin injections.

There are other measures of your health. Albumin is a protein that can be a measure of your nutritional status. If albumin levels in the blood are too low, you will need to eat more calories and protein. Even if you are eating the recommended amounts of protein, you must consume sufficient calories from other sources, or your body will begin to burn protein for fuel. In addition, your nephrologist will assess your liver function as a general health measure and to look for toxicity from any of the medications that you take.

I recommend that you monitor and understand all of your laboratory results. Your nephrologist or dialysis nurse can teach you the meaning of excessively higher or lower values and tell you about any treatment changes that might be required if the laboratory results change. Learn how to manage your diet, lifestyle, and compliance to your dialysis regimen. You may want to keep copies of the results to help you get a sense of what is optimal for you. All of these steps will give you more control over your health and well-being.

Pros and Cons

Each type of dialysis has advantages and disadvantages. Talk to your nephrologist about these pros and cons to decide which type is best for you.

Peritoneal Dialysis

Only 8.2 percent of patients choose or are able to use peritoneal dialysis. The main advantage of peritoneal dialysis is independence, because it does not require trips to a dialysis unit. Peritoneal dialysis works best if you are a self-starter, disciplined, and physically able to perform the necessary steps involved. Peritoneal dialysis is a better treatment than hemodialysis for people with low or unstable blood pressure (which can make hemodialysis difficult or even hazardous), a bad heart, or poor vascular access to the blood supply. Peritoneal dialysis gives you more control over when, where, and how exchanges are performed. Depending on your work situation, you may be able to dialyze in your office without interruption. Having a private space during exchanges can make peritoneal dialysis the more attractive option. You can even dialyze in the car if you have a long drive ahead of you. Avoid exchanges in public bathrooms or other places where contamination is a greater possibility.

Peritoneal dialysis also requires fewer dietary restrictions than hemodialysis. However, the body loses a lot of protein during peritoneal dialysis. You may need to take a protein supplement. One drawback of protein supplements is that many of them contain high levels of phosphorus, especially if they come from dairy products. One excellent option is powdered egg whites, sold by Optimum Nutrition at www.optimumnutrition.com, which taste good and mix well with water, milk, or juices. Your local GNC store may carry this product or can order it for you. If you have diabetes, you may have trouble controlling your blood sugar with peritoneal dialysis, since the dialysate contains glucose. Talk to your nephrologist about the potential nutritional side effects of peritoneal dialysis.

If you like to travel or must travel often for your job, peritoneal dialysis may be preferable to hemodialysis. Dialysis bags and other treatment tools can be sent directly to your hotel. (Contact your equipment supplier in advance to make arrangements for delivery.) When traveling by plane, people who use CCPD can place the cycler in the overhead bins, as long as they are physically capable of handling a 30-pound machine. Because checked luggage can be lost, it is a good idea to carry extra caps and tubing in your carry-on luggage. For travel within the United States, the Americans with Disabilities Act protections should allow a traveler to take a dialysis machine onboard the plane, but with today's strict airport security procedures, you should always check with the Transportation Services Administration before traveling with your dialysis equipment. For international travel, contact the airlines.

There are some disadvantages that may dampen enthusiasm for peritoneal dialysis. Peritoneal dialysis can be time-consuming and disruptive (although CCPD is less so). You must perform dialysis every day, regardless of your activities. Generally, you should be able to integrate exchanges into your life. However, depending on your work or travel schedule, you may have to arrange to do dialysis in the company of strangers, which you may find embarrassing. Occasionally, you can skip an exchange, which is not a disaster as long as you rarely do so. Remember, you will feel your best if you perform all of the exchanges that your nephrologist prescribes.

Although not as common as in the past, infections like peritonitis are still possible. If you live in an area where the water supply comes from an unchlorinated well, or if you have any concerns about recurring infections and showers, whether using city or well water, you should consult your doctor for advice. Also, be diligent about cleaning your exit site using a sterile cotton swab dipped in a special bleach solution your dialysis nurse will provide. These precautions should minimize your chances of getting peritonitis. If you do get peritonitis, you might need to spend one or more days in the hospital getting treatment. Peritonitis is treatable, but if you have recurrent episodes, you may need to have your catheter removed.

Peritoneal dialysis also causes weight gain and an increased waistline, which are mostly caused by fluid retention. It may be difficult to find clothes that fit properly, because your abdomen may become quite large. Moreover, you may feel uncomfortable with the dialysate pressing against your abdomen, especially if you have polycystic kidney disease (PKD) and large kidneys. If you have PKD, your nephrologist will help you to determine if peritoneal dialysis is a good choice for you.

If your home has limited storage space, you may have trouble storing your boxes of dialysate and paraphernalia. In addition, carrying heavy bags of solutions can be difficult, especially if you are weak from the disease and have no one to help you on a daily basis. If you are single and live alone, peritoneal dialysis may not be for you.

Peritoneal dialysis also requires dealing with a considerable amount of waste. The empty boxes, some of which do not collapse, can create a special challenge if you do not have municipal curbside trash removal. Some people must transport their trash to a local disposal site. If you have to haul your own trash, you will need to transport it more often, especially if you do not have a large vehicle. If you cannot remove your trash regularly, the amount of discarded material can become overwhelming. You may need help from your family or friends to manage the trash problem.

Peritoneal dialysis offers many advantages if you prefer to be responsible for and manage your own treatment. Although it can be very time consuming, peritoneal dialysis offers enough benefits that it may work well for you. Talk to your nephrologist and share your interests and concerns. She will be able to help you make a decision that will be best for you.

Hemodialysis

Hemodialysis has some advantages. For example, it is a good choice for people who like to spend time around other people. In addition, hemodialysis treatments provide structure and a consistent schedule to follow, with technicians at a center taking care of you. All you have to do is show up, and the nurses and technicians do the rest.

At hemodialysis centers, patients often develop a sense of camaraderie with other patients and the technicians. Because you will be spending so much time with these people, it helps if everyone is on good terms. You may even develop some close relationships at the dialysis center and they help pass the time. Some patients like talking, whereas others just prefer to sleep and be left alone. Or they watch television, read, or work on a laptop. In some dialysis centers, the social worker organizes activities and exercise programs.

The disadvantages of hemodialysis are related to the advantages. Although people may prefer having a flexible schedule for their dialysis treatments, people with full-time jobs may not be able easily to schedule treatments. The stress of commuting, especially in a large metropolitan area, just adds to the difficulty of traveling to a dialysis center. For those living in rural communities, travel distances to a dialysis center may be long. Getting to and from a dialysis center can be a problem if you do not drive. Public transportation and taxicabs are options, and many people have relatives and friends who are happy to help with transportation. But care-givers run the risk of burning out while they try to help a loved one and find their own schedules becoming overburdened. The social worker at the dialysis center can assist you with finding suitable transportation if you need it.

Medically, too, hemodialysis has a disadvantage that peritoneal dialysis does not have. As we saw previously, hemodialysis is an intermittent form of dialysis. Unlike peritoneal dialysis, which continuously dialyzes patients, hemodialysis allows waste products and imbalances in blood chemistries to accumulate between sessions. As a result, you will have to monitor your fluid, potassium, and phosphorous levels carefully. As with the peritoneal catheter, the access for hemodialysis may become infected.

Other disadvantages of hemodialysis involve the procedure itself. Because your vascular access, whether a fistula or graft, is penetrated with needles, you may experience discomfort or pain. If you need it, ask the technician to use a local anesthetic, like lidocaine.

During or after hemodialysis, you may develop cramps in your legs or feet, or you may feel lightheaded when you try to stand up. These symptoms are due to excess fluid removal during sessions, which is needed because you consumed too much fluid between sessions. The best solution is to restrict your fluid intake. Some dialysis centers will give you a salty solution to drink after a session. Although that helps at the time, you may feel thirstier and drink more fluid later. If you have difficulties restricting your fluid intake, talk to your dietician about strategies to help you. You might try avoiding having drinks close by or sucking on ice chips when you are thirsty. I found not having drinks nearby to be a particularly useful strategy in restricting fluid intake. When working and keeping my mind otherwise engaged, I successfully kept my intake to 1 liter per day.

Complications related to the access may also develop over time, including clotting, infections, and bleeding. Your nephrologist can manage most of these side effects. If a fistula or graft develops a blockage, then an interventional radiologist will be called in to remove the blockage. She will insert a catheter into a major vein in the groin, snake it into the fistula or graft, and attempt to dislodge the obstruction. If the blockage is a blood clot, the radiologist may use an enzyme called thrombin plasminogen activator (TPA) to dissolve it. Or she may insert a balloon, which can be inflated to enlarge the interior of the access site. Sometimes radiologists cannot repair the fistula or graft, and the patient will need a new access.

DIET

Fluid and dietary restrictions are more difficult to manage with hemodialysis than they are with peritoneal dialysis. This is especially true for controlling sodium, potassium, and phosphorus.

Excess salt (sodium) retention (and therefore fluid retention) is often the most difficult to manage. Salt is in almost everything we eat, and sodium levels are especially high in processed foods and restaurant foods. Thus, knowing how much sodium you are consuming becomes critical. Here is what happens if you ingest too much salt.

The body uses salt (sodium chloride) to keep a balance between the volume of blood and the volume of fluid in the tissues. The proper balance is essential for healthy hydration. Ingesting too much salt has several consequences. The sodium draws water from cells in the bloodstream and into the tissues outside of cells. This can raise the volume of blood and can contribute to hypertension. The overfilled tissues swell, causing fluid retention in the legs and feet. In addition, excess fluid in and around the lungs can cause shortness of breath. Excess salt ingestion also stimulates thirst, which can lead a person to drink too much fluid, causing fluid overload in the body. You can minimize fluid retention by strictly controlling both your salt intake and your fluid intake. For some people the nephrologist will establish a limit of 1 liter (approximately 1 quart) of fluids a day.

Potassium levels in the blood must be prevented from rising too high. The best way to control potassium levels is by restricting potassium in your diet. High potassium concentrations in the blood can lead to heart spasms and potentially death. Therefore, limit high-potassium foods, like orange juice, bananas, tomato paste, potatoes, and colas. See table 6.1 for a complete list of foods to avoid. Table 6.2 lists foods with low amounts of potassium.

High phosphorus levels have long-term implications—unlike high sodium and potassium levels, which pose more immediate concerns. As we learned in chapter 4, high phosphorus can lead to weakened bones and to the formation of plaques in various organs. Avoid foods that are high in phosphorus (see table 6.3). Take phosphate binders if your nephrologist prescribes them. Table 6.4 suggests how to substitute food with low phosphorus levels for foods with high levels.

Read food labels to identify potentially harmful ingredients. Consider getting a nutritional guide to some of the foods you commonly eat. The American Association of Kidney Patients offers a free guide on their website, which includes sodium, potassium, phosphorus, protein, and caloric values (see www.aakp.org).

You may feel overwhelmed at first by the list of dietary dos and don'ts. A dietitian can help you avoid the wrong foods, while showing you how to continue eating some of the foods you love. Restricting your diet may be difficult at first, but when you begin to feel so much better, you will decide it is worth it. Over time, tracking food values becomes second nature.

Table 6.1
Foods with High Levels of Potassium

Fruits	Vegetables	Other Foods
Apricot, raw	Acorn squash	Bran/bran products
(2 medium), dried	Artichoke	Chocolate (1.5–2 oz)
(5 halves)	Baked beans	Granola
Avocado (1/4 whole)	Bamboo shoots	Milk, all types (1 cup)
Banana (1/2 whole)	Beets, fresh then	Molasses (1 tbsp)
Cantaloupe	boiled	Nutritional supplements:
Dates (5 whole)	Black beans	Use only under the
Dried fruits	Broccoli, cooked	direction of doctor or
Figs, dried	Brussels sprouts	dietitian
Grapefruit juice	Butternut squash	Nuts and seeds (1 oz)
Honeydew	Carrots, raw	Peanut butter (2 tbsp)
Kiwi (1 medium)	Chinese cabbage	Salt substitute/lite salt
Mango (1 medium)	Dried beans and peas	Salt-free broth
Nectarine (1 medium)	Greens, except kale	Snuff/chewing tobacco
Orange (1 medium)	Hubbard squash	Yogurt
Orange juice	Kohlrabi	
Papaya (1/2 whole)	Legumes	
Pomegranate (1 whole)	Lentils	
Pomegranate juice	Mushrooms, canned	
Prunes	Parsnips	
Prune juice	Potatoes, white and	
Raisins	sweet	
	Pumpkin	
	Refried beans	
	Rutabagas	
	Spinach, cooked	
	Tomatoes/tomato	
	products	
	Vegetable juices	

Source: National Kidney Foundation website at www.kidney.org.

Note: Each item listed is a 1/2-cup portion, unless otherwise stated, and contains 200 milligrams or more of potassium.

The healthier your diet is, the fewer complications you are likely to have. Eating right requires self-discipline and understanding from your family and friends, who must be sensitive to your dietary needs, since you may not be able to eat what they serve. At times, you may have cravings for foods that you should not eat. You may find that you can *occasionally* eat these foods, but do so spar-

Table 6.2
Foods with Low Levels of Potassium

Fruits	Vegetables	Other Foods
Apple (1 medium)	Alfalfa sprouts	Bread and bread products
Apple juice	Asparagus (6 spears)	(not whole grains)
Applesauce	Beans, green or wax	Cake: angel, yellow
Apricots, canned	Cabbage, green and red	Coffee: limit to 8 oz
in juice	Carrots, cooked	Cookies (no nuts or
Blackberries	Cauliflower	chocolate)
Blueberries	Celery (1 stalk)	Noodles
Cherries	Corn, fresh (1/2 ear),	Pasta
Cranberries	frozen (1/2 cup)	Pies without chocolate or
Fruit cocktail	Cucumber	high-potassium fruits
Grape juice	Eggplant	Rice
Grapefruit (1/2 whole)	Kale	Tea: limit to 16 oz
Grapes	Lettuce	
Mandarin oranges	Mixed vegetables	
Peaches, fresh	Mushrooms, fresh	
(1 small), canned	Okra	
(1/2 cup)	Onions	
Pears, fresh (1 small),	Parsley	
canned (1/2 cup)	Peas, green	
Pineapple	Peppers	
Pineapple juice	Radishes	
Plums (1 whole)	Rhubarb	
Raspberries	Water chestnuts,	
Strawberries	canned	
Tangerine (1 whole)	Watercress	
Watermelon (limit to	Yellow squash	
1 cup)	Zucchini squash	

Source: National Kidney Foundation website at www.kidney.org.

Notes: Each item listed is a 1/2-cup portion, unless otherwise stated, and contains less than 200 milligrams of potassium. If you eat higher amounts of an item than stated, you risk converting it into a high-potassium food.

ingly and in small quantities. You may find that you need only the taste of these foods to feel satisfied. Stick to your basic diet (see chapter 5) and avoid forbidden foods and you will probably be okay. Be honest with your dietitian and nephrologist about what you are eating, especially if your blood chemistries are abnormal. They will be able to help you modify your diet to keep you healthy and allow you to eat some of the foods you like.

Table 6.3
Foods with High Levels of Phosphorus

	Beverages	
Ale	Chocolate drinks	Drinks made with milk
Beer	Cocoa	
Canned iced teas	Dark colas	

	Dairy Products	
Cheese	Custard	Pudding
Cottage cheese	Ice cream	Yogurt
Cream soups	Milk	

	Proteins	
Beef liver	Crayfish	Oysters
Carp	Fish roe	Sardines
Chicken liver	Organ meats	

	Vegetables (dried beans and peas)	
Baked beans	Kidney beans	Pork 'n' beans
Black beans	Lentils	Split peas
Chickpeas	Lima beans	Soybeans
Garbanzo beans	Northern beans	

	Other Foods	
Bran cereals	Nuts	Whole grain products
Brewer's yeast	Seeds	
Caramels	Wheat germ	

Source: National Kidney Foundation website at www.kidney.org.

Note: A high-phosphorous food generally has more than 100 milligrams per serving.

RESTLESS LEGS SYNDROME

People undergoing hemodialysis may experience restless legs syndrome. Estimates of the percentage of people affected range from 6 to 60 percent of people having hemodialysis. *Restless legs syndrome,* a neurological disease with an unknown cause, is a strong urge to move the legs that is difficult to resist. Patients describe restless legs syndrome as creepy-crawly, itching, pulling, tugging, or gnawing sensations. These sensations begin when the person is at rest, not moving, and especially when going to sleep. The symptoms of

Table 6.4

Low-Phosphorus Substitutions for High-Phosphorus Foods

High-Phosphorus Foods (mg phosphorus)		Low-Phosphorus Substitutes (mg phosphorus)	
8 oz milk	230	8 oz nondairy creamer	100
		4 oz milk	115
8 oz cream soup made with milk	275	8 oz cream soup made with water	90
1 oz hard cheese	145	1 oz cream cheese	30
1/2 cup ice cream	80	1/2 cup sherbet or 1 Popsicle	0
12 oz can cola	55	12 oz can of Ginger Ale or lemon soda	3
1/2 cup lima or pinto beans	100	1/2 cup mixed vegetables or green beans	35
1/2 cup custard or pudding made with milk	150	1/2 cup pudding or custard made with nondairy creamer	50
2 oz peanuts	200	1 1/2 cup light salt/low fat popcorn	35
1 1/2 oz chocolate bar	125	1 1/2 oz hard candy, fruit flavors or jelly beans	3
2/3 cup oatmeal	130	2/3 cup cream of wheat or grits	40

Source: National Kidney Foundation website at www.kidney.org.

restless legs syndrome can be extremely unpleasant. You may have an uncontrollable urge to move and jerk your legs. If you resist it, the negative feelings may be overwhelming, almost painful. Moving may be the only way for the sensations to stop. Ultimately, you may get little sleep and feel exhausted during the day.

Treatments are available to relieve the symptoms of restless legs syndrome. To determine whether these treatments are right for you, your nephrologist will first examine your nutritional status. Deficiencies in iron and certain vitamins, like B-12 and folate, can contribute to restless legs syndrome. However, since most people on dialysis take iron and vitamin supplements, nutrition is usually not the cause of restless legs syndrome for them.

Various medications can help relieve the symptoms of restless legs syndrome. For people with chronic kidney failure, low doses of a drug like clonazepam (Klonopin), which is a benzodiazepine derivative with anticonvulsant, muscle relaxant, and anxiety-relieving properties, may provide relief. Other drugs in this same class may give you a hangover, however. Clonazepam works very well, even using the lowest dose needed to alleviate the symptoms. If you have restless legs syndrome, treatment with clonazepam may help you get a good night's sleep and feel rested during the day.

Anticonvulsants are another class of drugs your nephrologist may prescribe. Originally developed to treat Parkinson's disease, anti-convulsants like pramipexole (Mirapex) and ropinirole (Requip) may be helpful in treating restless legs syndrome. The downside is that anticonvulsant drugs have caused nausea, lightheadedness, and, in rare cases, hallucinations in some people taking these medications to treat Parkinson's disease. Since treating restless legs syndrome requires lower doses of these drugs than for Parkinson's disease, the side effects may not be as severe.

If you have restless legs syndrome, talk to your nephrologist. You do not have to suffer from this disorder.

No one likes dialysis, and it is neither risk free nor complication free. However, it is possible to make dialysis tolerable and to limit how much it interferes with your activities. Talk about your options with your nephrologist, and understand your own temperament and lifestyle. If you cannot obtain a transplant from a living donor before going on dialysis, the waiting time for kidney transplants can be long. Help yourself during this time by complying with your treatment, following your prescribed diet, restricting your fluid intake, and taking your medications. Taking care of yourself will make dialysis tolerable and will keep you in the best health possible.

A successful kidney transplant may be your best chance at living a long and healthy life. That's the topic of the following chapter.

7

TRANSPLANTATION

We live in a consumer society. We buy things and we throw things away, sometimes with little thought. But many people are developing a greater awareness that discarded items pile up in landfills, and as a result they are taking steps to recycle and reuse materials when they can.

Many people now view organ transplantation the same way. People who might otherwise die because of organ failure can live longer lives through *transplantation* of organs from living or deceased donors. Surgeons can transplant kidneys, livers, hearts, lungs, pancreases, intestines, bowels, bone, tendons, veins, corneas, and skin.

Organ transplantation has come a long way over the last thirty years. In the early years of transplantation, doctors thought they could only transplant a viable organ from one person to another if the donor and the recipient were identical twins—otherwise, the recipient's body would reject the donated organ. Modern medicine has made major advances in the techniques of transplantation, and new drugs have been developed that suppress the body's normal reaction of rejecting a foreign body. How does transplantation work? How is it even possible? This chapter explores these questions and explains the transplantation process.

When medical science gained an understanding of how the immune system fights off foreign invaders, it was able to develop treatments to prevent organ rejection. For example, scientists used this knowledge to create vaccines to help the body destroy specific invading organisms like those that cause polio. The vaccines helped the body produce proteins, called *antibodies*, which attack the invading organisms and cause their death. But even without a vaccination, the healthy immune system dispatches an army of cells to kill many bacteria, viruses, and other microorganisms it encounters that do not belong in our bodies. The healthy immune system is pretty amazing. But here's the downside for people who need transplants: because the body considers transplanted organs to be foreign, the immune system will attack them.

The body has an ingenious way of knowing what belongs to it and what does not: every cell in a person's body possesses a marker— a "nametag" of sorts—that distinguishes it from the cells in another person's body. When cells with different nametags bump into each other, a series of reactions occur, sometimes leading to the destruction of the cells that do not belong.

These nametags are known as *antigens*. Inside the body, cells called *lymphocytes* recognize whether the antigen belongs to you or to someone or something else. If your lymphocytes encounter recognizable cells, nothing happens. However, if your lymphocytes do not recognize a cell's antigens, the invading cells are killed. In the case of organ transplants, a specialized lymphocyte called a T-lymphocyte destroys the organ. When we are talking about transplantation, we refer to the degree to which the cells are compatible with one another, and therefore the nametags relevant to transplants are called histocompatibility antigens, or human leukocyte antigens (HLA).

Your *HLA typing* and the HLA typing of the donor define how compatible a donor kidney may be. Only six of the many histocompatibility antigens must be known before your compatibility for a kidney transplant from another person can be evaluated. These six antigens come in more than one hundred forms and are not equally present in the population. Some are more common than others. The most common HLA antigens are present in about 20 percent of the population, whereas others are present in less than 1 percent of the population. In addition, some HLA antigens provide a stronger immune response than others do. These variables mean that finding a similar match from someone outside your family can be difficult.

Until recently, for a transplant to succeed, these antigens had to be closely matched. Now, because researchers have developed more effective anti-rejection drugs, an antigen match is less important than it once was. A perfect match is still best, but less than perfect matches can be managed almost equally well with the latest immunosuppressant medications.

Are You a Candidate?

Kidney transplantation is the treatment of choice for kidney failure, allowing for the best quality of life. Your nephrologist will determine whether you are eligible to receive one. A kidney transplant is a serious operation, and living with a transplanted kidney requires lifelong care. Any donated organ is a valuable gift that must be given only to people who will take care of it. Therefore, you must take all prescribed medications, keep your doctors' appointments, and take care of yourself.

Your nephrologist will assess whether you will be a responsible transplant recipient based on your previous behavior. For example, if you are on dialysis, your nephrologist will find out whether you came to the dialysis center for all of your treatments (or performed all of your prescribed exchanges, if you are on peritoneal dialysis). In addition, he will check that you have taken all your medications and complied with any prescribed dietary restrictions. With a new kidney, your quality of life will improve, but that does not mean that your health is no longer an issue. After all, a transplant is not a cure for kidney failure; it is only a treatment. Thus, if your nephrologist does not think that you will be compliant, he will not recommend you for a transplant.

Several other conditions can make it difficult to receive a transplant. Because the immune system will be deliberately suppressed with medications after a transplant, you cannot have an active infection or uncontrolled infectious disease, like a bacterial infection, at the time of the transplant. If you are HIV positive or have hepatitis B or C, you can receive a transplant, but complications are more likely. To be eligible for a transplant, you must not have cancer or smoke. Evidence of drug or alcohol abuse will prevent you from getting a transplant until the problem has been resolved. Obesity may also exclude you from receiving a transplant. Although the policies of transplant centers vary, your potential longevity will be assessed to determine whether you would benefit from a transplant, especially if you do not have a living donor. The waiting time for a deceased donor may be years, so your likely future condition will be taken into consideration.

On a happier note, many people do qualify as transplant recipients. The prospect of receiving a transplant can be very exciting, especially if you have been on dialysis for a long time. Your ability to work, to engage in activities you love, and to just feel normal again will improve with a successful transplant. This chapter covers the steps you will take if transplantation is an option for you.

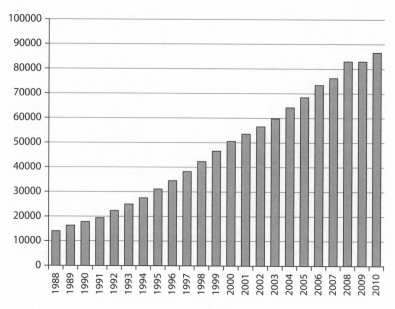

Figure 7.1. Number of Transplant Candidates on Waiting List, 1987–2010

Donors

The number of people receiving kidney transplants has been steadily increasing since 1987. Ever since kidney transplantation began, there have been fewer kidney donors available than the number of kidney donors that are needed (as we saw in chapter 1). As of October 2010, according to the United Network of Organ Sharing (UNOS), over 86,000 candidates in the United States were waiting for kidney transplants, continuing this trend (see figure 7.1). In 2009, 16,829 people received kidney transplants, down from a high of 17,095 in 2006 (see figure 7.2).

Kidneys come from two types of donors: living donors and deceased donors. As we learned above, not enough kidneys are available and acceptable for transplantation. This means long wait times

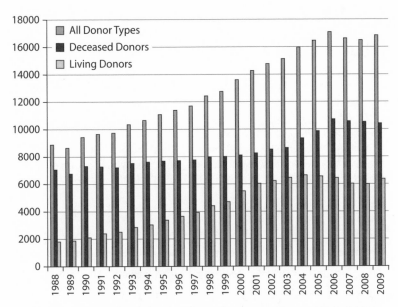

Figure 7.2. Number of Transplants by Donor Type, 1988–2009

for many patients. This is especially true for people with type O blood, the most common blood type, because so many type O potential recipients exist for donations from type O donors. Survival rates for kidney recipients from both living and deceased donors are quite good. Table 7.1 displays the one-year, three-year, and five-year kidney survival rates as well as patient survival rates for people who received a kidney from living donors versus those from deceased donors. (Kidney survival means living without dialysis or another transplant.) Patient survival is better than kidney survival, because patients may go back on dialysis after losing a kidney while they wait for another transplant.

Another way to measure survival is using the half-life. The half-life is the time that represents 50 percent of those surviving kidneys that reach that point. The half-life of a kidney from a living donor is 20 to 25 years, while the half-life of a kidney from a deceased

Table 7.1
Kidney Transplant Survival Rates

	Living Donor		Deceased Donor	
	Kidney	Patient	Kidney	Patient
1 year	95.1	97.9	89.0	94.4
3 years	87.8	94.3	77.8	88.3
5 years	79.7	90.1	66.5	81.9

Source: United Network for Organ Sharing website at www.unos.org. Data are derived from transplants performed 1997–2004, compiled as of March 13, 2009.

Note: One-year survival is derived from 2002–2004 transplants, three-year survival on 1999–2002 transplants, and five-year survival on 1997–2000 transplants.

donor is 7 to 10 years. Thus, half of people receiving a kidney from a living donor will still have that kidney functioning for 20 to 25 years, and half of people receiving a kidney from a deceased donor will still have that kidney functioning in 7 to 10 years.

Living Donors

The public is more aware of the need for organ donations than ever before and, as a result, more people are promising to donate their organs when they die. However, many organs are needed *now* to save the lives of people whose organs have failed. New interest in living donation has given hope to many patients in need of a kidney transplant. Since 1988, according to UNOS, the total number of living donations steadily increased, peaking in 2004. The number of living donations has been steady since then (see figure 7.2). As a percentage of kidney transplants, living donations also increased, until peaking at almost 43 percent in 2003 and then declining to 38 percent in 2009 (see figure 7.3). The decline in living donations as a percentage of all kidney transplants is a result of the rapid swelling in the number of people needing transplants, as well as of an increased availability of more usable organs from deceased donors.

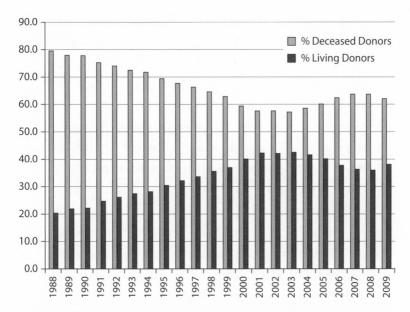

Figure 7.3. Percentage of Transplants by Donor Type, 1988–2009

Kidneys received from living donors generally have better success rates than those received from deceased donors. You may want to find a person willing to donate a kidney to you—although approaching someone about a living organ donation may be awkward. After all, you are asking someone to give up a body part, risking her own health and with no medical benefit to her. Therefore, the gift has to be truly altruistic. One approach to finding a donor is making your circumstances known to your family, friends, or groups you are involved in. If someone is interested in donating a kidney to you, he or she will approach you.

Another source of donations is a kidney pool. In recent years there has been an increase in the number of individuals donating kidneys to a non-directed pool of recipients through organizations like the New England Program for Kidney Exchange (NEPKE), MatchingDonors.com, and the National Kidney Registry (see the

Resources section at the end of the book). In donor pools like these, anonymous or "Good Samaritan" donors do not specify the person receiving the transplant. To ensure that their gift is suitable, donors must be thoroughly screened and educated about the potential risks. Moreover, they must not be compensated for their donation, since cash payments for organ donations are illegal in the United States. If donations to a non-directed pool become more common, they could help relieve the imbalance between the number of organs available and the number of organs needed.

If you are tempted to buy a kidney abroad, do not do it! Studies have shown that people who do so generally have poorer outcomes. Because the donors *are* motivated by money, they may not be well screened medically. Medical tourism has become a flourishing business; marketing practices now include the temptation of exotic vacations coupled with a transplant from a living donor. Don't be fooled: *it is not worth the risk.* If you have a family member or friend living abroad, however, that opportunity may be worth pursuing as long as the donor is thoroughly screened and as long as it is a good match. Explore this possibility only through reputable transplant centers abroad. Talk to your local transplant center for advice.

Although many direct kidney donations from loved ones have good outcomes, a potential donor may not be compatible, usually because of an unacceptable blood type or a preexisting disease like polycystic kidney disease (PKD). In an attempt to increase living donation, better methods have been devised to screen and match donors and recipients, so that more transplants might be possible (see the Resources section for details).

If you find a willing donor but that person is not a suitable match, you may be able to take advantage of a system of swapping, commonly called a paired kidney donation. Here is how it works. If you have an incompatible donor, your transplant center will try to locate another transplant candidate whose incompatible donor is compatible with you. If your donor is compatible with the other candidate, you can swap donors. If the second donor is not compatible with you, your transplant center may try to find other candidate-donor pairs where one donor is compatible with you, and their incompatible donors are compatible with the other candidates. In such a case, a more complex candidate-donor swap can be performed. A Good Samaritan donor can even initiate a chain of donations if he or she is compatible with a candidate who does not have other compatible donors available.

With today's advances in removal and transfer of a kidney from a living person, most surgeons can remove a donor's kidney laparoscopically. In laparoscopic removal, the surgeon makes small incisions in the abdomen and then extracts the kidney through one of the incisions. The other incisions allow the surgeon to insert a video camera and surgical instruments. A minimally invasive laparoscopic operation means quicker recuperation for the donor than in traditional removal methods, which require an incision under the rib cage and which can cause greater discomfort and longer recovery times.

When you are ready for a transplant, the transplant team will organize a meeting with your donor, whom you may or may not have already met, to explain the process and to answer any questions about living donation, the surgical procedure, and the short-term and long-term risks associated with a donation. These meetings may include family and friends. All information gathered about the patients and the procedure is confidential. Your transplant team may separate you and your donor for counseling and examination. Your donor will be seen by a nephrologist different from yours for the workup. Your donor and you will also have different surgeons. Medicare now requires that every program have a living donor advocate who is available to talk to your donor about concerns or reservations. Medicare and most medical insurance plans cover the cost of testing the donor for compatibility.

Both you and your donor will undergo extensive physical examinations, be asked to provide your medical histories, and will undergo a battery of tests performed by your respective medical teams to ensure that your kidneys are compatible and that donating a kidney will not adversely affect the donor's health. In addition, your donor's nephrologist will make sure the donor does not have kidney disease and that he or she has two kidneys; the donor's nephrologist will rule out any infectious disease or cancer risk that the donated kidney may pose to you. If there are warning signs of potential pitfalls at any point in the process, your donor can opt out.

The team will discuss with you, the recipient of a transplant, what's involved in your surgery, what will take place during the hospitalization, and what you will need by way of follow-up care after you are discharged from the hospital. A crucial part of your aftercare is the medications you will need to take to help your body resist rejecting your new kidney and becoming infected by various microorganisms. Therefore, the transplant team will discuss your ability to pay for your medications, which can be very expensive, to make sure that you have adequate insurance or other financial means to cover their costs. Medicare will cover most of the costs of medications for three years after surgery, but for now (legislation is pending in Congress to remove the three-year limit) other health insurance policies or personal funds will be needed to cover the rest of the cost for the first three years and most of the cost after that.

In most cases you and your donor must have compatible blood types, although some centers have transplanted blood-incompatible candidates on an experimental basis. Because of the way we inherit blood types, some blood types are compatible and some are not

Table 7.2
Blood Type Compatibility

Donor	Candidate
A, O	A
B, O	B
A, B, AB, O	AB
O	O

(see table 7.2). For example, if you have type O and your donor has type A, B, or AB, your immune system will reject your donor's kidney. Thus, you both must have type O blood. On the other hand, if you have type A, B, or AB, you can accept a kidney from your donor not only if he or she has the same blood type, but also if he has type O. Type O is known as the universal donor. If you have type AB, you can accept your donor's kidney regardless of his blood type, making type AB a universal acceptor.

Other blood tests will assess your and your donor's general health, and can reveal whether either of you has any active infections, including hepatitis or HIV/AIDS. An electrocardiogram (EKG) and stress test will be done to assess the activity and function of the heart, to rule out underlying cardiac conditions that might endanger the health of you or your donor during or after surgery. Any condition that could harm your donor's remaining kidney, like high blood pressure or diabetes, would disqualify him as a candidate. Finally, a social worker will conduct an interview with your donor to assess whether the kidney is being donated for the right reasons and not in exchange for payment or some other compensation.

Deceased Donors

Organs may also be obtained from a recently deceased person (cadaver). Not surprisingly, organs from deceased donors are more difficult to match to recipients than living donations are. With more people needing kidney transplants than there are kidneys available, the U.S. government, through a contract with UNOS, has established what it believes is a fair and equitable procedure to allocate and match kidneys.

According to its website (www.unos.org), UNOS coordinates organ transplantations of all types with the transplant centers throughout the United States. UNOS also coordinates multiple-organ transplants, like kidney/pancreas and heart/lung. As of October 2010, UNOS maintained a database for all organs of more than 108,930 people needing an organ. UNOS oversaw 28,464 transplants in 2009.

The UNOS database helps match organs from deceased donors to appropriate candidates. When kidneys become available, the organ procurement team removes them and sends information about the blood and tissue types via computer to UNOS, where staff members match potential candidates on the waiting list. Using the blood type, size of the organ, the patient's time on the waiting list and medical urgency, as well as the geographic distance between the donor and patient, the computer generates a list of potential candidates.

The transplant coordinator in the transplant center then contacts the transplant surgeons caring for these patients. Each kidney has one primary recipient and at least one backup recipient. Because time is crucial, the transplant center is required to spend only one hour trying to contact the primary and backup candidates before UNOS goes to the other candidates on the waiting list. To minimize the time between recovering a kidney from a donor and placing it in a candidate, UNOS divides the United States into eleven regions (see figure 7.4).

When a candidate on the waiting list matches perfectly with an available donor kidney, that candidate goes to the top of the na-

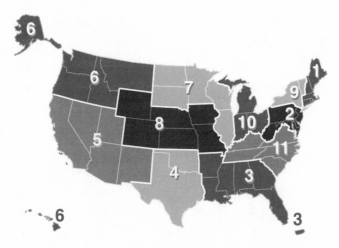

Figure 7.4. The Eleven National Regions of the United Network of Organ Sharing

tional list regardless of how long he or she has been on the list. About 20 percent of transplants from deceased donors are a perfect match. When no candidate matches perfectly with the available donor kidney, UNOS offers the kidney first to a candidate with the next best match living in the same locality, and then living in the same region, before offering it to the rest of the country. Additional consideration is given those under 25 years old and highly sensitized individuals (those who have had previous transplants, transfusions, or pregnancies, in the case of women) because these conditions introduce foreign cells into the candidate, increasing the chances of rejection. Furthermore, some kidneys are transplanted along with a heart or a liver to the candidate when the person has kidney failure as well as severe heart or liver failure.

Although a candidate's chances of receiving a transplant improve the longer he is on the list, candidates do not actually occupy a particular slot. Ranking occurs only when a kidney becomes available. Until recently, the primary consideration for a transplant depended on the extent to which the HLA type of the candidate matched the HLA type of a donor with the same blood type. Now, a perfect match still goes to the top of the list, whereas with kidneys for which there is no perfect match on the waiting list, the time a candidate has spent on the waiting list is a predominant criterion.

Unlike candidates receiving transplants from living donors, where there are options for blood type compatibility, an organ from a deceased donor must be an exact match. Requiring an exact match provides fairness for people with a particular blood type. Giving kidneys from donors with type O blood to people with other blood types, while possible, would create a greater shortage than exists now for type O candidates, meaning an even longer wait time, which is currently the longest for all candidates. Therefore, it is not done. Once an exact blood type match is established, the cells from the deceased donor and from the candidate undergo further testing.

There are two classes of kidneys from deceased donors: standard criteria donors and expanded criteria donors. Expanded criteria donors differ from standard criteria donors by age and medical condition. Any donors over 60 years old are considered expanded criteria donors. Expanded criteria donors also include people over 50 years of age with any two of the following characteristics: high blood pressure, heart attack or stroke, diabetes, or a blood creatinine over 1.5 mg/dl. An expanded criteria donor may be an option for people with complications that may make it impossible for them to wait very long for a transplant. However, kidneys from expanded criteria donors typically do not function well in the beginning and may have a shorter survival.

The best candidates for an expanded criteria donation are people with diabetes over the age of 40 and people over 50 whose blood supply is difficult to access for dialysis. Candidates on the waiting list may receive transplants from an expanded criteria donor sooner than receiving one from a standard criteria donor. If an expanded criteria donor interests you, talk to your nephrologist and transplant team to find out whether it is an option for you under your medical circumstances.

Elderly people may want to consider an expanded criteria donor, although their general eligibility for a transplant will depend largely on their overall health status. A nephrologist will assess the benefits and risks of a transplant to assess whether transplantation would increase their lifespan and quality of life, compared with staying on dialysis. Because kidneys from expanded criteria donors may not initially function normally, recipients must be healthy enough to tolerate both dialysis and the effects of immunosuppression. Their nephrologist will help them decide if a transplant is appropriate for them at that stage of life.

Before any transplant, laboratory tests will be done to assess the likelihood that the candidate's immune system will reject the transplanted organ. One test compares the *Panel Reactive Antibody (PRA)* of the donor and the candidate. PRA measures the amount of antibodies in the blood as a way of assessing the probability of rejection. With a high PRA, chances of rejection increase. These antibodies, which can sensitize a kidney to rejection, can be present as a result of previous transplants, blood transfusions, a disease like lupus, or pregnancies.

The other test is the cytotoxic *crossmatch*, where lymphocytes from the deceased donor are mixed with the candidate's blood to determine whether antibodies are produced in the candidate's blood that could cause immediate rejection of the kidney. A positive crossmatch indicates certain rejection. Thus, a *negative* crossmatch is desired. Once these criteria have been satisfied, the transplant surgery can proceed.

UNOS is currently developing a new system for allocation that will make better use of transplanted organs, matching kidneys with people who have the greatest expected survival time. As of this writing, the system has not gone into effect. Check the UNOS website, www.unos.org, or consult your transplant team for updates.

Waiting for a Transplant

The wait for a kidney transplant can be frustrating and can seem endless.[1] Many people with kidney failure decide to get a kidney transplant rather than start or continue dialysis. After undergoing all the extensive tests and finally being placed on the transplant list, the wait begins. For a lucky few, the wait is short. Some people receive transplants within months. However, most people wait for years for a transplant. For people who have not found a compatible kidney from a living donor, the wait is about three to seven years. Wait times also vary depending on where in the country a candidate lives. I was on the list for more than seven years, and the wait was often difficult.

When I first started dialysis, I was quite ill. I didn't think much about transplantation until I became well enough to consider it. Then my biggest concern was being unavailable to my transplant coordinator who could call at any time to say, "It's time." Like many people on the wait list, I carried a cell phone; I also had a pager with me at all times, not knowing whether I would receive a signal when in a large building or far away from home.

The longer I was on the transplant list, the less I wanted to travel very far from home. Wherever I went, I made sure the transplant coordinator knew where I was and how she could contact me. Even so, I was always concerned about receiving a call or returning in time to receive my kidney. Although a surgeon can effectively transplant a kidney within twenty-four hours, the chances that the kidney will function immediately decrease with increasing time after removal from the donor. Consequently, I lived in fear that I would miss that great gift of life by being in the wrong place at the right time.

Those of us on the transplant list know that we have limited ability to plan for the day the transplant coordinator calls. We could have a bag packed and have family and friends ready to help, but we do not know for sure if our plans will work. It is not as if we know exactly when our transplant will happen. Over the seven and a half years I lived with dialysis, although I often found myself becoming increasingly anxious about my availability for a transplant, all I could do was stay in contact with the hospital, hang in there, live my life the best way I could, and wait. Although patience may be a virtue, at times I found it hard to maintain. At some point, we need faith that in the end, everything will work out. We will receive our transplant, and our lives will improve.

Having a Transplant

When the time comes for your transplant, it is often a surprise. Many candidates waiting for transplants receive numerous calls that do not pan out. Because UNOS does not know for sure whether the primary candidates are available, many candidates receive calls as possible backups to determine their readiness. Eventually, you will percolate to the top of the list and finally get your call as a primary candidate.

Once you receive the call and accept the organ, you will go to the transplant center to prepare for surgery. The center will perform blood tests to make sure your health is good enough for the transplant surgery to proceed. Part of waiting for surgery involves the time to transport the kidney to the center and to complete the crossmatch to ensure that you will not reject your new kidney immediately. As one of the final preparations for surgery, a nurse will insert a catheter into a vein, and the anesthesiologist will begin administering sedatives. Once in the operating room, the anesthesiologist will give you general anesthesia.

The transplant itself, whether the kidney comes from a living or deceased donor, is relatively simple, as figure 7.5 illustrates. In living donations, left kidneys are transplanted because they have longer *ureters* (the long tubes connecting the kidney to the bladder) than right kidneys. In deceased donations, either kidney may be used. The organ procurement surgeon dissects the kidney from the deceased donor and its attachments from its surroundings. The kidney is immediately perfused with a preservation solution composed of high potassium and other nutrients and is cooled down to decrease oxygen demand; these steps keep the kidney as healthy as

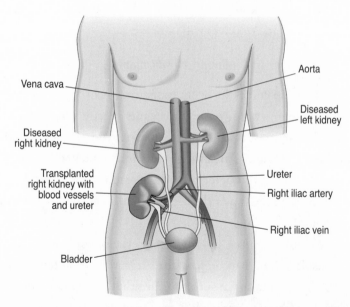

Figure 7.5. The New Kidney in Place after the Transplant Procedure.
The transplanted kidney on the right side of the body appears on the left in the figure, which is facing us.

possible. In the operating room, your transplant surgeon will place the kidney into your lower abdomen. He or she will attach the blood vessels of the new kidney to the external iliac artery and vein in the groin, and then attach the new ureter to the bladder. During the operation, the surgeon will insert a Foley catheter into the urethra to the bladder to collect urine. The old kidneys are not usually removed unless they are chronically infected, as in PKD patients with infected cysts. Otherwise, they don't normally pose a threat to the patient.

Postoperative Care

After the three- to four-hour transplant operation, proper care and monitoring becomes essential to manage postoperative pain, to prevent rejection of your kidney, and to minimize infections. Your recovery in the hospital will last, on average, five to seven days, during which time you will receive numerous medications to control the aftereffects listed above. Initially, your immune system must be heavily suppressed with anti-rejection medications, which reduces the likelihood of rejecting the organ but increases the likelihood of contracting infections. To counteract this possibility, you will receive antibiotic, antiviral, and antifungal agents to reduce the chances of infection. You must take these medications exactly as prescribed. Before the transplant you will have told your transplant team about any other medications you are taking, and the team will make adjustments in medications to avoid potentially serious drug interactions.

Once released from the hospital, you must keep daily records of your blood pressure, temperature, fluid intake, and urine output, and have your blood tested regularly to detect the possibility of infection or kidney rejection. You must also eat a healthy diet and exercise regularly once your incision has healed. A healthy lifestyle is essential during the first year (and beyond) to keep your body in the best shape possible. The post-transplant coordinator at the center will outline the regimen you must follow. The need for blood tests diminishes over time, as your body accepts the new kidney.

Taking immunosuppressants over the longer term is the cornerstone of treatment to prevent rejection of your newly transplanted kidney. Your transplant surgeon, depending on the center's protocol and experience, can prescribe several different drugs. Before and immediately after the transplant, intravenous medications like anti-thymocyte globulin (Thymoglobulin), daclizumub (Zenapax), and basilixamab (Similect) may be administered to reduce the chances of rejection. The main anti-rejection medications currently prescribed for long-term use are steroids like prednisone (Deltazone), methylprednisone (Medrol), tacrolimus (Prograf), sirolimus (Rapamune, Rapamycin), mycophenolate mofetil (Cellcept), mycophenlic acid (Myfortic), and cyclosporine (Neoral, Gengraf). Cheaper generic medications may be available; if you desire to use them, talk with your transplant team, who must approve the use of generic medications.

An estimated 10 to 40 percent of transplant recipients experience acute rejection during the first six months post-transplant. However, with time, the body accepts the kidney and the doses of immunosuppressants will be reduced to maintenance doses. If acute rejection does occur, short-term treatment with high doses of immunosuppressant medications is administered, and adjustments will be made to the maintenance doses of these drugs. If acute rejection occurs numerous times, the kidney may undergo chronic rejection by the body, which can lead to the loss of function over the long term.

Immunosuppressant drugs have many side effects. Because they suppress the immune system to prevent rejection, the body becomes more prone to infections of all types, including bacterial, viral, and fungal infections. During the first six months after transplant, im-munosuppression is at its highest level. To reduce the risk of infec-tion during this time, doctors will prescribe separate drugs for each threat, like sulfamethoxazole/trimethoprim (Bactrim) for bacterial infections like pneumonia, acyclovir (Zovirax) for viral infections like herpes, valganciclovir (Valcyte) for cytomegalovirus (CMV), and clotrimazol troche (Mycelex) for fungi, especially of the mouth and throat. If you have no infections after six months, your surgeon will discontinue these medications.

Immunosuppressants may increase your risk of developing can-cer, especially lymphoma. People taking immunosuppressants are also at a higher risk of developing skin cancers. Careful monitoring is required to detect cancer early and to initiate early treatment. The monitoring for cancer includes periodic assessments of whether levels of viruses, normally under control by the immune system, are elevated. This is especially true for the Epstein-Barr virus, which can cause lymphomas. You will need regularly scheduled diagnostic tests like mammograms, PAP smears, colonoscopies, and skin can-cer screens to prevent cancers from developing out of control.

Another side effect of anti-rejection medications is developing elevated blood lipids (*hyperlipidemia*), which are higher than normal values for cholesterol and triglycerides in the blood. Elevated cho-lesterol and triglycerides are risk factors for heart disease and stroke. If you have elevated blood lipids, you will need to take a drug like atorvastatin (Lipitor), simvastatin (Zocor), or fenofibrate (Tricor). In addition, you must eat a low-fat diet.

Steroids pose additional complications for transplant patients. As we have seen throughout this book, diabetes is the major cause of kidney failure. Unfortunately, both steroids and tacrolimus can complicate management of Type 2 diabetes. People who do not have diabetes are at risk of developing the disease while taking steroids. Steroids may also increase your risk of developing osteoporosis. Osteoporosis results from the loss of calcium from the bones, making them more brittle and prone to fracture. If you have been on dialysis, you are probably familiar with this risk, which steroids may only increase. Fortunately, many transplant centers are now prescribing steroids less. At some centers, doctors eventually wean their patients off steroids altogether.

People awaiting a transplant are at a higher risk of developing hypertension because blood pressure may be difficult to manage. After a transplant, it is common for blood pressure levels to decline dramatically. However, some immunosuppressants can elevate blood pressure, as well as increase the risk for cardiovascular disease. Your center will closely monitor your blood pressure for any sudden increases or decreases.

Weight gain is a common problem with those receiving a transplant. In some cases, the weight gain can be as much as 100 pounds. This is caused by the immunosuppressant medications. Not only do some of them lead to fluid retention, they can also inhibit the ability of the body to burn fat deposits. Although you will be able to eat whatever foods you like, you may find that you will have to limit your caloric intake. I have had this problem since I had my transplant. To deal with weight gain, in addition to limiting my food intake, I engage in a rigorous, daily exercise program consisting of strength training and aerobics that keeps my weight under control. As an added benefit, this program has also kept my blood pressure and blood glucose levels under control without the need of any medications. Before you start such an exercise program, consult your transplant team to ensure that you are physically able to do it.

Because the functioning of one transplanted kidney will never be equivalent to two normal kidneys, your creatinine, blood urea nitrogen (BUN), and glomerular filtration rate (GFR) will be monitored. If kidney function begins to deteriorate after many years, your nephrologist will assess whether any of the health problems that you experienced before your transplant, like anemia and bone disease (see chapter 4), are similar to the current decline.

In spite of potential complications after transplant, with a new kidney you can expect a considerable improvement in your quality of life. You should have no problem working, traveling, and engaging in the activities that you enjoy. You may find, as many transplant recipients do, that receiving a kidney transplant is like being born again. You will feel so much better that in time you may forget the worst experiences of kidney failure. Life will be yours for the taking, but only *as long as you care for your new kidney and follow all of the instructions of your transplant team*. Remember, a kidney transplant is not a cure but a treatment.

Clinical Trials

Participating in a clinical trial is one route to receiving a transplant. Clinical trials are research projects using human subjects and are designed to answer specific health questions. Most trials assess whether a new medication or procedure will be an effective treatment for patients with a specific disease. In the case of kidney transplants, numerous clinical trials are under way. To learn more about them, visit the National Institutes of Health (NIH) Clinical Trials website at www.clinicaltrials.gov.

I became interested in clinical trials more than a year before I received my kidney transplant, when I realized that receiving a new kidney might not be the end of living with kidney failure. I could be unlucky and lose my kidney to rejection or infection. Therefore, I decided to focus on finding ways to maximize the long-term success of my new kidney and to reduce the possible complications induced by immunosuppressant drugs by possibly enrolling in a clinical trial designed to do just that.

After talking to my transplant coordinator and the social worker at my dialysis center, I learned that NIH had ongoing clinical trials that matched my interest. I called the transplant coordinator at NIH and told her of my interest in participating in a trial. After thoroughly reading the research protocols, I made an appointment to meet with the transplant coordinator and the principal investigator.

The goal of my first visit was to gather information about the program and the credentials of the researchers. Being a researcher myself, I wanted to delve into the scientific rationale of their research, their accomplishments and disappointments with their results, and the possible risks of enrolling in the trial. I scoured the publications that they provided.

The science behind their research and the trial made a great deal of sense to me. The researchers designed the protocol to make the body tolerant to the presence of a foreign organ, thereby reducing the likelihood of rejection. In doing so, a transplant recipient would need fewer immunosuppressant drugs to avoid rejection. As to risk, they had lost no kidneys due to rejection since NIH established their transplant institute in 1999. Only two kidneys were lost because of viral infections.

Knowing these statistics, I decided that I could accept the risks and that the clinical trial was worth considering seriously. From what the doctors told me, I was convinced that participating in the trial would not adversely affect the outcome, compared to standard care at a traditional transplant center. As additional insurance, I asked my nephrologist to call the principal investigator, who was also the transplant surgeon, to assess for herself the potential risks I would be taking. After talking to the surgeon, my nephrologist felt that I would not be taking any additional risks if I participated. After doing my own research and with the support of my nephrologist, I decided to enroll in the study and did not look back. My preparation for the transplant I received through the clinical trial mirrored the preparation described earlier in this chapter.

More than six years have passed since my transplant, and I have experienced no rejection episodes and no significant infections. I am currently taking a small dose of only one immunosuppressant drug. Moreover, I no longer have high blood pressure. As a result of living a healthy lifestyle, I have been able to travel all over the world, which is what I enjoy doing.

After participating in this clinical trial, I arrived at several conclusions about the benefits and drawbacks of clinical trials, and I have some ideas about how to decide whether to participate in one. Here are some issues to consider.

How Far Along Is the Research?

Clinical trials progress in several phases based on the number of subjects and the questions asked. Phase I trials tend to have fewer participants and are designed to determine the safety of the medication and range of doses for use in future trials. If the medication is new, with few studies done in humans, the greatest risk could occur during Phase I trials. Other Phase I trials are designed to test drugs approved by the Food and Drug Administration (FDA) for one application, but researchers want to evaluate their use for a new application, perhaps for a disease for which the medication was not originally intended. In this case, participation in a Phase I trial is less risky, because much of the drug safety testing has already been done.

Phase II trials enroll more subjects, typically a few hundred. At this stage, efficacy and safety become important factors. I chose to participate in a Phase II trial because the experimental drugs had already been FDA approved for another application. In addition, the researchers had good evidence that the protocol had a high chance of success.

Phase III trials may involve thousands of patients, and are conducted in multiple centers around the country and even the world. By this point, safety and efficacy have been reasonably established. The risks are substantially reduced, but death or less severe complications may occur in a small percentage of participants.

Understanding the Protocol

Scientific research is often difficult to understand, especially for people who do not have training in science. The scientific jargon can sound like a foreign language. Although I understood much of it, there were terms and research issues that were unfamiliar. Anyone participating in a clinical trial has the right to understand fully what the study involves and what risks are possible. Keep asking questions until you are satisfied that you understand all of the potential risks and rewards. If necessary, ask your doctors for help. I found that my nephrologist's input helped allay any remaining concerns I had about enrolling.

Advancing Medical Research

Many people decide to enroll in a clinical trial because conventional means of treatment have not been successful. Their participation in a clinical trial may be their only hope for survival. Good candidates for kidney transplants typically do not face this dilemma. Standard transplant protocols are acceptable and are generally preferable to remaining on dialysis.

Even in clinical trials, the use of medications or procedures occurs only after rigorous research, first with experimental animals and then with human subjects. To advance this research, human volunteers are needed. If people did not participate in clinical trials, there would be no new drugs! People who participate in clinical trials realize that they are making a significant contribution to improving the health of their fellow humans and perhaps themselves, too. The prospect of making a difference gave me considerable satisfaction. I had worked in medical research for more than thirty years, and my participation gave me an opportunity to continue contributing. You may feel the same way.

Medical Insurance and Care

Another benefit of enrolling in a clinical trial is cost. People who enroll in a trial receive free treatment and health care relevant to the study, which may be especially attractive for people who do not have medical insurance. Although Medicare will cover much of the cost of a transplant, the remaining costs can still be substantial. A transplant recipient can save a considerable amount of money, especially for prescription drugs, by participating in a trial. Even though I had a good health insurance policy, participating in the clinical trial still saved me money.

My Experience

My transplant surgeon called me at 3:30 one morning to tell me that my time had come to receive a new kidney. I was happy yet apprehensive about what to expect. Even though I had prepared for this day, now the idea of a transplant changed from the abstract to a reality.

At 6:30 a.m., I drove to NIH, where for several more hours I waited for the lab to complete the final testing to make sure I was compatible with the kidney. At about 11:00, the nurse placed an intravenous line into my arm and gave me a sedative. As the nurses wheeled me down to the operating room, the sedatives must have kicked in, because I do not recall getting there. I awoke several hours later in the recovery area with a new kidney.

For me, the immediate postoperative issues were recovering from the anesthesia and managing pain. I find general anesthesia disorienting. In the past, I have had visual and sometimes auditory hallucinations for several days after receiving general anesthesia. Although I found this disconcerting, I knew that they would go away. An additional complication for me was getting my bowels to function properly, which took several days. Pain can be managed with a morphine drip or by self-administration using a pump, which controls the amount, maximum dose, and appropriate intervals of intake. (Morphine, unfortunately, tends to cause constipation, which further complicates the bowel problem.) Thanks to a morphine drip, I had no significant postoperative pain, even though I had an eight-inch incision in my lower abdomen.

As part of the clinical trial, I received a medication just after my transplant to further reduce my chances of rejecting my kidney. In addition to anti-rejection medications, my doctors prescribed anti-thymocyte globulin (Thymoglobulin) for several days to deplete the T-cells responsible for rejection. This treatment kept my T-cell count low for almost two weeks. In the program's experience, the immune systems of patients given anti-thymocyte globulin were less responsive to a foreign kidney, compared to a standard treatment protocol. For me, anti-thymocyte globulin had a strange side effect. My hands itched, and then the skin peeled. They were unsightly for a while, but they returned to normal after the last dose of the drug.

Before transplant, my high blood pressure was difficult to control, even with high doses of three different blood pressure medications. After my transplant, my blood pressure dropped to the point where I needed only one medication. After six months, I no longer needed any blood pressure medication at all. More closely controlled blood pressure was a major benefit of having a kidney transplant.

Like many people receiving kidney transplants, I had elevated blood lipids before receiving a transplant. In fact, my blood lipids were initially so high after my transplant that the nurse who drew my blood could see the fat in the sample. It was fortunate that I did not have a heart attack or stroke. At the time, I was taking sirolimus and tacrolimus as my anti-rejection medications. To treat the high blood lipids, my doctors took me off the sirolimus, which was identified as the cause. With proper treatment—in my case, with fenofibrate (Tricor), pravastatin (Pravachol), and fish oil capsules—I have maintained normal blood lipid levels.

Another complication I experienced was contracting the Epstein-Barr virus. Although the level of the virus was high, I had no symptoms. Still, my doctors were concerned enough to call in a specialist on the virus to examine me. In his opinion, I required no specific treatment, but my doctors were instructed to monitor the virus carefully. Because they believed that the elevated level of the virus suggested that I was excessively immunosuppressed, they decided to lower my doses of anti-rejection medications.

Reducing the amount of immunosuppressants I was receiving could have placed my kidney at risk of rejection. In my case, lowering the dose of my medication not only reduced the level of the virus but also lowered my blood creatinine. If my body were rejecting my kidney, my blood creatinine would have risen. Because anti-rejection drugs can damage the kidney, less immunosuppression actually helped in my case.

My experience with a clinical trial may not be typical. Being part of an experimental program to reduce the amount of immunosuppression needed, rather than getting a transplant under standard care, probably reduced my risk of rejection owing to viral infections.

A friend of mine died from complications of lymphoma resulting from a high degree of immunosuppression. In his case, he lost his kidney and passed away after a dialysis treatment. This was another reason why I chose to enroll in the clinical trial.

Six months after my transplant, I no longer had to take the antimicrobial medications and took only a low dose of tacrolimus as my immunosuppressant. At that point, I felt great and started creating my new life. To determine whether a clinical trial is right for you, consult your nephrologist for help.

As we learned earlier in the chapter, kidney transplantations have very high rates of success. Most of the transplant recipients whom I know personally, regardless of whether they received them through a standard protocol or a clinical trial, have responded very well to their new organs. Some had complications, but they eventually healed and are enjoying life to the fullest. So can you. If you have no significant complications after your transplant, you, too, can live a normal life, and kidney failure can become a distant memory.

8

FUTURE
TREATMENT OPTIONS

Throughout this book I have discussed treatments that are currently available for people with kidney failure. I have also discussed options for treating the causes of kidney failure. This chapter looks ahead to what the future may hold in terms of new treatments for people with failing kidneys.

In the 1950s, when my mother confronted kidney failure caused by polycystic kidney disease (PKD), there were no treatments for hypertension, anemia, or kidney failure itself. Neither dialysis nor transplantation was readily available for people with kidney failure from *any* cause. At the time, kidney failure was a death sentence.

Over the last five decades, however, dedicated research has yielded many new treatment options for people at risk for kidney failure. Not all of these new treatments are optimal, and their side effects sometimes impede quality of life. For example, although kidney transplantation is the treatment of choice for kidney failure, the availability of a donor kidney is uncertain, and the underlying disease might take its toll while the person is waiting for a transplant. In addition, once a transplant has been performed, the side effects of immunosuppressant drugs can be life threatening. If the prospect of kidney failure is in your future or in your children's future (that is, if your family has a strong genetic predisposition for kidney failure), looking ten to twenty years ahead, at how the next generation might fare, may give you hope about the future of treatment. Although some of this discussion is speculative, the prospects are plausible. Only time will tell if any of these promising new approaches to treatment come to fruition.

New Medications

The Human Genome Project, which sequenced the genes on each of the twenty-three human chromosomes (see chapter 3), may allow scientists to find the proteins that each gene makes. With a comprehension of the role of these proteins in operating the biochemical reactions of our cells, we may begin to understand the underlying defects that cause disease. Research is under way to identify potential targets, like receptors or enzymes involved in an abnormal response. Once the targets have been identified, researchers can develop new medications to work effectively with those targets.

Historically, developing a medication involves studying its overall effectiveness and safety in a *population* of people with a disease, because not all people react to the drug in the same way. In study populations, responses vary, and researchers use analytical tools to decide whether a drug will be useful and safe in the clinic *on the average*. Because many genes could be involved with a disease, the response to a specific drug by a specific patient could be different from how the *average* person reacts to the drug; for example, the patient may react differently on the basis of the drug target or the way the patient's body processes the drug.

In the future, doctors may be able to predict how an individual will respond to treatment, resulting in individualized health care that is tailor-made to a person's specific characteristics, not just to how people on average respond to a medication. In the future, health care treatments may be modified on the basis of a person's genetically mediated responses to a number of medications, some of which may be effective and some not. This new approach to treatment is called *pharmacogenetics*. Depending on the condition, this promising future treatment could analyze a person's genetic code to determine whether her genetic attributes support the use of a particular treatment.

Pharmacogenetics may also yield information about the target of the medication and how the body breaks down the drug. For example, the liver metabolizes drugs using enzymes, which have different activities, based on the variants of the genes involved. Identifying which genetic variants of liver enzymes a person has could help doctors prescribe drugs that are most likely to work according to that person's genetic makeup.

Although in its infancy, pharmacogenetics has already led to the development of better treatments for some diseases. It has been known since the 1950s that certain genetic variants in a number of enzymes that metabolize drugs in the liver can enhance or reduce their effectiveness. More recently, the treatment of hepatitis C has been greatly improved by the observation that a protein known as artificial interferon is more effective in patients with a particular genetic variant than in people without it.

Whether a pharmacogenetic approach will yield improved treatments for kidney disease remains to be explored. A better understanding of the mechanisms underlying different diseases is more valuable for treating some illnesses, but not all. Because a specific disease can be associated with many variations in the genetic code, as is the case with diabetes, any specific variation might contribute a great deal—or very little—to the expression of the disease. Thus, pharmacogenetics holds the most promise with diseases in which there is variation of only a few genes contributing to the expression of the disease.

Individualized treatment based on a person's genetic code is not a far-fetched idea. The cost of performing the sequencing has plummeted dramatically in recent years. Sequencing one person's complete genome will probably cost as little as $1,000 or possibly less in the future. In the future, too, sequencing a child's entire genome at birth may become a routine procedure. Because a person's genome does not change over time, it would be necessary to sequence each person's genome only once, and therefore this would be a one-time expense. In the future, as we begin understanding how and when genes turn on and off, it may be possible to determine which genes are overactive or underactive in a disease state and to tailor the treatment to the process that a specific gene mediates. Currently it is possible in diseases like cancer to predict the response to a particular form of treatment based on a certain genetic characteristic of the patient.

There is a downside to genome sequencing and to knowing a person's predispositions to specific diseases. For one thing, a predisposition to a disease does not necessarily mean a person will get the disease. Many diseases develop only when a person who has the genes that make him susceptible to the disease encounters something in the environment, like a virus, which turns the disease "on." Some critics argue that genetic sequencing could cause people to worry needlessly, because they might never develop a disease, even though their genes indicate that they have the *potential* to develop the disease. There is also some concern that worried individuals will get unnecessary medical procedures to monitor for disease. Also, evidence that a person is at risk for a specific health condition might lead insurers or employers to discriminate against that person. In an effort to combat this concern, the Genetic Information Nondiscrimination Act was signed into law in 2008; this Act specifically forbids such discrimination on the basis of genetic information. In addition, the passage of the Patient Protection and Affordable Care Act in 2010 will prohibit this type of discrimination beginning in 2014.

Dialysis

People who have been on dialysis know that it is an often unpleasant treatment for kidney failure. Although dialysis keeps us alive and can improve our quality of life, it can be uncomfortable and has numerous other drawbacks. As we learned in chapter 6, both peritoneal dialysis and hemodialysis have their pros and cons.

Peritoneal dialysis allows us to perform our own treatment but can be inconvenient in terms of where we can perform exchanges. In addition, peritoneal dialysis causes weight gain and loss of protein, and carries the risk of peritonitis. Hemodialysis must be performed on a specific schedule that may not be convenient, especially considering the demands of employment. People on hemodialysis may experience side effects like lightheadedness, nausea, bleeding from the fistula or graft, and infections. To have hemodialysis, a person must take a great deal of time out of his normal schedule to make clinic visits several times a week. Regardless of what form of dialysis we choose, the drawbacks can take a toll.

Currently under study and in use in some centers is an approach involving more frequent hemodialysis treatments. Current practices for hemodialysis require dialysis three times a week, either in a center or at home. Because intermittent dialysis is less efficient than continuous dialysis, newer approaches involve shorter, more frequent (daily) treatments.

A variation of this approach is nightly home hemodialysis, in which patients dialyze while they sleep using a slower flow rate, with a typical treatment lasting seven hours. Proponents of nightly home hemodialysis claim that patients maintain better control of their blood chemistries, have fewer problems with anemia, have better blood pressure control, and spend less time in the hospital.[1] The current number, organization, and location of technicians and nurses may not be adequate to process the increased workload of daily treatments, even though this approach might benefit many patients. Currently, Medicare and health insurance companies do not routinely cover these techniques, but extra treatments might be justified on the basis of improved patient outcomes. Another drawback to nightly home hemodialysis is that it can be difficult to secure the needles in the access to avoid serious and potentially life-threatening bleeding.

Also under development are wearable hemodialysis machines to allow for more frequent dialysis.[2] These designs use small mini-pumps and dialyzers but have sorbent systems, which absorb the dialysate and clean and recirculate it, reducing the need for a large fluid source. Still in the early stages of development, wearable hemodialysis units have the potential to increase the quality of life of patients by improving their medical outcomes and reducing the amount of time they spend in dialysis centers.

Finally, artificial filters or dialyzers that are more efficient might improve the medical results of hemodialysis. Because the crux of hemodialysis is the dialyzer, improving its filtering capabilities, while sparing the integrity of red blood cells and reducing stress on the body, could improve medical outcomes for patients. Some newer dialyzers are better able to retain protein and remove excess phosphate. Perhaps dialyzers of the future will be even more effective.

Transplantation

Receiving a kidney transplant is a great gift of life, whether you were on dialysis or were fortunate enough to get a new kidney before your kidneys completely failed. The freedom that a transplant gives is immeasurable. Being able to return to my normal activities made a great difference in my quality of life. Although you must take medications for the rest of the useful life of your kidney, it is far better than being tethered to a dialysis machine.

As we saw in chapter 7, the biggest risk associated with organ transplants is rejection. Because the body perceives the new kidney as a foreign invader, the immune system will attempt to destroy it. Therefore, as part of the post-transplantation care regimen, transplant recipients take drugs that suppress the immune system. The immune-suppressing medications available today are quite good in preventing rejection. However, there are serious potential side effects. A suppressed immune system increases the risks of contracting infections and some forms of cancer. Some of these conditions can be life threatening. In addition, the risks of developing diabetes, cardiovascular disease, and osteoporosis increase, especially when taking steroids.

A possible solution to these complications may be the development of immunosuppressants targeted to the part of the immune system responsible for rejection. Now, physicians use medications that suppress *all* cell-mediated immune functions. In the future, new drugs might target immune functions that relate only to transplanted organs. That approach would put much less stress on the body.

Another approach currently under study but not yet widely used is lowering the response of the immune system to the presence of a foreign organ. I participated in such a study when I received my transplant (see chapter 7). The premise involved depleting the cells that cause rejection—T-cells—for about two weeks, which allowed enough time for my body to get used to the new kidney. As a result, I needed far less immunosuppression than is usually required, thereby reducing my risk of developing the complications that often result from the standard protocol. With further research, this approach could be tailored to the individual patient. Eventually, it may be possible to avoid rejection all together.

One intriguing line of research, called *xenotransplantation*, involves assessing whether kidneys from animals (like pigs, which have kidneys that are structurally similar to human kidneys) could be used as donors for human transplant. Although it would seem almost certain that the recipient's body would reject the kidney from another species, scientists hope one day to genetically engineer pigs so the pigs' kidneys are immunologically less reactive or inactive in a human patient. Another difficulty with xenotransplantation is the risk that the animal's organs might contain retroviruses that could infect a recipient. Further research will be needed to find out whether xenotransplantation will be a viable treatment for kidney failure in the future.

Stem cells may prove to be another promising avenue to improving the success rates of transplantations. Stem cells, when they are in the right form, can transform into any cell type in the body under the proper conditions; thus, stem cells someday may be used to grow new body parts, including kidneys, for people who need them. Stem cells can come from either embryonic cells (from human embryos or human umbilical cord blood) or adult cells. Although researchers are studying stem cells as precursors for making specialized cells to correct many diseases, the moral implications of using embryonic stem cells have hampered research for this purpose.

Adult stem cells, especially when they are taken from the same person who needs treatment, have great appeal in the treatment of disease. However, adult stem cells have not yet shown their promise as being a good substitute for embryonic stem cells. Recent studies were performed that successfully converted adult human cells to embryonic stem cells and then delivered them to the correct targets using viruses.[3] Unfortunately, however, the embryonic stem cells had high rates of cancer development. In very recent research, scientists were able to avoid using a virus and successfully converted the adult cells into an embryonic state.[4]

Even if either embryonic or adult stem cells can be manipulated to make any type of cell we want, we know very little about the complex process the body uses to create an organ from those cells. During fetal development, various genes turn on and off at various times to construct each organ. As one can imagine, the prospect of re-creating the organ development process outside the womb is daunting, as it would require taking skin cells or other types of cells from a person needing a new organ, like a kidney, converting the cells through a series of steps into a kidney, and then transplanting it into the patient. Because the kidney would be genetically identical to the patient, no immunosuppression would be required. Only time will tell whether such an approach to transplantation will ever be possible.

Scientists are pursuing all of these different avenues of research at the same time. Anyone who reads the newspaper or listens to radio or watches television knows that breakthroughs in medical treatment happen all the time. One day a new edition of this book will be needed, because the treatment of kidney disease will have advanced so far that current treatments are outdated.

I look forward to writing that new edition.

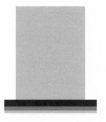

EPILOGUE

I t can be devastating to receive a diagnosis of failing kidneys. It can be daunting to anticipate what lies ahead, including the difficulties of treatment. Educating yourself about the decisions you must make, as well as using all the tools available to you, will help you manage the process. Ultimately, it will be up to you to decide how hard kidney failure will be for you.

Throughout this book I have emphasized the importance of taking responsibility for your health. Accepting that you are primarily responsible for your health will empower you as you face the prospect of kidney failure.

You now have a great deal of information about how to prevent or postpone kidney failure. It is time to start implementing what you know. For some of you, the problem may seem far in the future, and perhaps secondary to the other priorities of life that compete for your attention. However, this is no time to be in denial. No priority is more important than your life. Without your health, nothing else will matter. I learned that lesson when my kidneys failed.

You have a choice: take action now, and prevent or postpone the problem, or suffer the consequences of inaction in the future.

Take control of your health. No one should be more motivated than you are to improve your future quality of life. Your family and friends can help you, but understand that they have only so much time and energy to lend. Find ways to help yourself and do not depend totally on others, not even your doctors. Your doctors may give the best medical advice, but they are not responsible for implementing their advice. *You are!* Use the advice in this book, and find ideas of your own that help you with your daily activities.

I know firsthand how tough it can be to take care of yourself when you are sick. With little energy, I had great difficulty even getting up in the morning, let alone taking care of routine, daily tasks. But on many days you will be well enough to do at least some of the most important things that require your attention. We all make occasional bad decisions or feel overwhelmed about our health situation. Try not to dwell on the setbacks. Celebrate your accomplishments and push aside your failures.

Kidney failure is a serious condition. But with commitment, patience, and practice you can make it. Along the way, create the life you want.

Remember:

Move quickly through denial and face your disease directly.
Be your own advocate.
Believe your life will improve.
Take the long view.
Remain optimistic and give a positive spin to everything.
Know your priorities and stick to them.
Be willing to take risks.
Ask for help, but don't depend on it.
Keep your sense of humor.

NOTES

Chapter 1 · UNDERSTANDING KIDNEY FAILURE

1. *U.S. Renal Data System, USRDS 2010 Annual Data Report: Atlas of End-Stage Renal Disease in the United States* (Bethesda, MD: National Institutes of Health, National Institute of Diabetes and Digestive and Kidney Diseases, 2010). Chronic kidney failure occurs in stages over many years. ESRD is the final stage and requires treatment, either dialysis or transplantation.

2. E. Kübler-Ross and D. Kessler, *On Grief and Grieving* (New York: Scribner, 2005).

Chapter 3 · WHY KIDNEYS FAIL

1. Obesity was measured by body mass index (BMI) weight in kilograms divided by the square of height in meters. A BMI greater than 25 is considered overweight, over 30 as obese, and over 40 as morbidly obese.

2. http://diabetes.niddk.nih.gov/dm/pubs/overview/index.htm.

3. D. Alshuler et al., "Genome-Wide Association Analysis Identifies Loci for Type 2 Diabetes and Triglyceride Levels," *Science* 316 (2007): 1331–1336; E. Zeggini et al., "Replication of Genome-Wide Association Signals in UK Samples Reveal Risk Loci for Type 2 Diabetes," *Science* 316 (2007): 1336–1341; L. J. Scott et al., "A Genome-Wide Association Study of Type 2 Diabetes in Finns Detects Multiple Susceptibility Variants," *Science* 316 (2007): 1341–1345.

4. M. A. Lazar, "How Obesity Causes Diabetes: Not a Tall Tale," *Science* 307 (2005): 373–375.

5. B. E. Wisse et al., "An Integrative View of Obesity," *Science* 318 (2007): 928–929.

6. G. Wolf and F. N. Ziydeh, "Molecular Mechanisms of Diabetic Renal Hypertrophy," *Kidney International* 56 (1999): 393–405.

7. A. B. Weder, "Genetics and Hypertension," *Journal of Clinical Hypertension* 9 (2007): 217–223.

8. T. Steinman, "Diagnosing PKD, Determining Options," *Nephrology News & Issues,* March 2006.

9. J. J. Grantham et al., "Volume Progression in Polycystic Kidney Disease," *New England Journal of Medicine* 354 (2006): 2122–2130.

Chapter 6 · DIALYSIS

1. *U. S. Renal Data System, USRDS 2010 Annual Data Report: Atlas of End-Stage Renal Disease in the United States* (Bethesda, MD: National Institutes of Health, National Institute of Diabetes and Digestive and Kidney Diseases, 2010).

2. This description is the one that I employed when on peritoneal dialysis using supplies provided by Baxter International, Inc. Supplies from other companies, like Fresenius, are also available.

Chapter 7 · TRANSPLANTATION

1. This section is adapted from an article I wrote for the PKD Foundation, "Waiting for a Kidney Transplant," *PKD Progress* 18, no. 2 (2003): 13.

Chapter 8 · FUTURE TREATMENT OPTIONS

1. A. S. Klinger, "More Intensive Hemodialysis," *Clinical Journal of the American Society of Nephrology* 4 (2009): S121–S124.

2. C. Ronco, C. A. Davenport, and V. Gura, "Toward a Wearable Artificial Kidney," *Hemodialysis International* 12 (2008): S40–S47.

3. J. Yu et al., "Induced Pluripotent Stem Cell Lines Derived from Human Somatic Cells," *Science* 318 (2007): 1917–1920.

4. J. Yu et al., "Human Induced Pluripotent Stem Cells Free of Vector and Transgene Sequences," *Science* 324 (2009): 797–801.

GLOSSARY

Acidosis   Buildup of acid in the blood.

Adrenal glands   Small endocrine glands sitting atop the kidneys that secrete aldosterone, promoting fluid and salt retention.

Albuminuria   Protein in the urine. Urine with high amounts of protein is called macroalbuminuria, while urine with low amounts is called microalbuminuria.

Aldosterone   See Adrenal glands.

Anemia   Low red blood cell count.

Aneurysm   Ballooning of a major blood vessel that can rupture, causing massive bleeding.

Angiotensin-converting enzyme (ACE)   Enzyme that stimulates the conversion of angiotensin I to angiotensin II.

Angiotensin system   System that regulates blood pressure when salt concentration is low; renin reacts with angiotensinogen, which stimulates the conversion of angiotensin I to angiotensin II, which then constricts blood vessels to raise blood pressure.

Antibody   A protein created by the immune system to attack and destroy foreign entities like microorganisms and organs transplanted from other people.

Antigen "Nametag" on cells that identifies the cells as belonging to a specific individual.

Atherosclerosis Buildup of plaque in blood vessels that can contribute to hypertension.

Autosomal dominant polycystic kidney disease (ADPKD) Dominant form of PKD; a child has a 50 percent chance of inheriting the disease from an affected parent.

Autosomal recessive polycystic kidney disease (ARPKD) Recessive form of PKD; a child has a 25 percent chance of inheriting the disease if both parents are carriers of the mutated gene, but the parents do not have ARPKD themselves.

Biopsy A procedure in which a small amount of tissue is removed from the body for investigation and testing.

Blood typing The means for determining one person's blood type compatibility with another person's blood type. Compatible blood typing is needed for kidney transplantation.

Blood urea nitrogen (BUN) A measure of kidney function. A high value indicates declining kidney function.

Bone marrow Soft tissue in bone that makes red blood cells.

Calcidiol An intermediate form of vitamin D in the production of calcitriol.

Calcitriol The most active form of vitamin D that the body uses. It does not require activation by the kidney and is often given to dialysis patients who cannot make their own calcitriol.

Calcium An important mineral in keeping bones strong and a mediator in many biochemical pathways.

Carbohydrates A group of sugars and starches that are a source of energy for the body.

Carbon dioxide The main substance in exhaled breath. In the form of bicarbonate, it neutralizes acidity in the blood.

Catheter Access to a major vein. Catheters are used primarily for dialysis but can be a means of administering medications or nourishment. They can also be used to drain urine from the bladder.

Cholecalciferol   The form of vitamin D typically found in supplements. Cholecalciferol does not have to be activated in the skin. See Vitamin D.

Chromosome   Structure within the nucleus of the cell that houses the genetic code. Each cell contains twenty-three pairs.

Continuous Ambulatory Peritoneal Dialysis (CAPD)   A form of dialysis that requires four to five manual exchanges of abdominal fluid per day.

Continuous Cyclic Peritoneal Dialysis (CCPD)   A form of dialysis that uses a machine (cycler) to perform exchanges during the night; some manual exchanges are needed during the day.

Creatinine   A measure of kidney function. Creatinine is completely filtered by the kidney, making it a more accurate measure than BUN. A high value indicates declining kidney function.

Creatinine clearance   The amount of creatinine filtered by the kidney and passed into the urine. This is the most accurate measure of kidney function.

Crossmatch   The last test performed to avert rejection of a donated kidney. A negative test result allows the transplantation to proceed.

Deoxyribonucleic acid (DNA)   Blueprint for life; DNA is composed of long strings of nucleotide sequences containing the instructions for making up to three proteins.

Diabetic nephropathy   Diabetes-induced kidney failure.

Dialysate   The solution drained from the abdomen during a peritoneal dialysis exchange; also, the solution bathing a dialyzer in a hemodialysis machine.

Dialysis   A method of cleansing the blood of waste products.

Dialyzer   A filter used in hemodialysis containing tiny filaments bathed with dialysate; blood passes through the filaments and toxins diffuse into the dialysate.

Edema   Accumulation of fluid in soft tissues of the body, especially in the legs and ankles.

Electrolytes   Salts, like sodium and potassium, which control many functions in the body.

Erythrocytes   Red blood cells, which carry oxygen throughout the body.

Erythropoietin (EPO)   A hormone made by the kidney to stimulate production of red blood cells (erythrocytes) in bone marrow.

Exchange   The process in peritoneal dialysis by which the dialysate is replaced.

Fistula   A vascular access created by joining an artery and a vein in an arm or leg, used for hemodialysis.

Genes   The instructions for making and running a cell; genes are composed of sequences of DNA.

Glomerular filtration rate (GFR)   A measurement similar to creatinine clearance, but calculated from blood creatinine taking into account age and race.

Glomerulus   A structure in the kidney that filters blood of its waste products.

Glucose   The main source of energy in the body.

Graft   A vascular access created by joining an artery and vein to each end of a Gortex tube, used for hemodialysis.

Hematocrit   The volume of blood comprising red blood cells.

Hemodialysis   Filtration of the blood with a machine that circulates blood through a dialyzer.

Hemoglobin   A protein in red blood cells that carries oxygen through the body. Hemoglobin levels can drop as kidneys fail.

Heparin   A blood thinner used in hemodialysis to avoid clotting in the tubing and dialyzer.

HLA typing   The means for determining one person's cells' immune compatibility with another person's cells. HLA typing is used for matching donors to recipients for a kidney transplant.

Homeostasis   The process of keeping conditions in the body within a normal range.

Hormones Substances, like aldosterone and leptin, acting on receptors that change physiological function.

Hyperlipidemia Elevated blood fats like cholesterol, saturated fats, and triglycerides.

Hypertension Blood pressure above 140/90.

Incidence The number of new cases of a disease.

Insulin A pancreatic protein that regulates glucose levels in the blood by helping glucose pass into cells.

Insulin resistance Reduced ability of insulin to enter cells, even when blood insulin levels are high.

Kidney failure A condition when elimination of wastes from the body no longer takes place.

Kt/V A measure of efficiency in hemodialysis.

Leptin A hormone that regulates hunger by reducing appetite; leptin may play a role in Type 2 diabetes.

Lymphocytes Cells within the immune system that protect the body from foreign organisms. T-lymphocytes attack transplanted organs, causing rejection.

Metabolites Substances formed through a series of biochemical reactions. For example, protein is broken down to urea.

Mutations Mistakes made in copying genes that can cause a malfunction in cellular processes and can lead to a disease like PKD.

Nephron The basic unit of the kidney, composed of a glomerulus, tubules, and collecting ducts.

Osteoporosis A condition in which excess amounts of calcium are removed from bones, making them brittle and more easily fractured.

Panel Reactive Antibody (PRA) A test to measure the amount of antibodies in the blood to assess the likelihood of kidney rejection. The higher the value, the greater the potential for rejection.

Parathyroid hormone　A hormone secreted from the two parathyroid glands in the neck that promotes removal of calcium in bone into the blood. This action can lead to osteoporosis.

Peritoneal dialysis　Filtration of the blood with a solution in the abdomen.

Peritoneal equilibrium test (PET)　A method to determine the adequacy of peritoneal dialysis by measuring the creatinine and urea in four hourly samples.

Peritonitis　Inflammation of the lining of the abdomen.

Pharmacogenetics　The use of genetic information to develop new medications. Specific mutations in genes and accompanied altered protein structure can suggest mechanisms underlying a disease that can be potential targets for therapeutic intervention.

Phosphorus　An important substance in the generation of energy. Phosphorus accumulates in hemodialysis patients and can combine with calcium in the blood to form plaques in organs, possibly leading to organ failure.

Polycystic kidney disease (PKD)　An inherited disease characterized by cysts that grow and ultimately destroy kidney function.

Polygenetic diseases　Diseases caused by mutations in multiple genes.

Potassium　A salt that helps regulate heart beat and brain function. High blood potassium levels can lead to heart block. Usually high potassium can be treated by altering the diet or prescribing medications.

Prevalence　The total number of people with a disease at a given time.

Proteins　Long chains of amino acids that operate cells and provide structure for the body.

Receptors　Entities on or within cells that translate a signal from a hormone or drug into a physiological response; receptors are specific for certain chemical structures, like a key fitting a lock.

Renin　A substance released from the kidney that activates the angiotensin system (see Angiotensin system). Under normal conditions it helps maintain blood pressure during dehydration or extreme blood loss.

Restless legs syndrome   A neurological disorder that can affect people on hemodialysis, who experience an uncontrollable urge to move their legs.

Sodium   A principal substance (salt) that determines how much fluid the body retains.

Transplantation   Organ replacement therapy where an organ is removed from one individual (a donor), either living or deceased, and placed in a recipient.

Urea   Breakdown product of protein. Urea is the main substance excreted by the kidney.

Uremia   Excess amount of urea in the blood, which can cause death in kidney failure patients without dialysis or transplantation.

Ureters   Long tubes that connect the kidneys to the bladder.

Urinalysis   A method used to detect blood or protein in the urine.

Urinary reduction rate (URR)   A measure of efficiency of hemodialysis.

Vasopressin   A hormone released by the pituitary gland that acts on the kidney to retain fluid.

Vitamin D   A fat-soluble vitamin needed to form and maintain strong bones. Vitamin D can be made naturally or supplied in the diet or with supplements. The kidney makes the most active form of vitamin D, and when kidneys fail, bone structure can degrade, requiring treatment with the most active form. This problem is most common in hemodialysis patients.

Xenotransplantation   Transplantation of an organ from one species to another.

RESOURCES

This resource list is for readers interested in learning more about kidney diseases, how the kidney functions, the diagnosis and management of kidney diseases, the principles of dialysis and kidney transplantation, and other topics not covered in detail in this book. Readers who wish to get involved in a community of patients and health care providers can use the list to identify and contact organizations whose sole purpose is to provide support to patients. Some of these organizations are advocates for patients and include congressional lobbying as part of their activities on behalf of patients.

The list of resources and organizations is not exhaustive but does include sources that I found most informative and authoritative.

EDUCATIONAL RESOURCES

The Internet is a seemingly unlimited source of information. Websites provide information and support, and scientific databases link to primary research articles on kidney diseases. The National Library of Medicine at the National Institutes of Health provides the best databases; see www.nlm.nih.gov. The most useful databases are PubMed and the NLM Gateway. PubMed is easier to use for simple searches; begin your searches at www.ncbi.nlm.nih.gov/PubMed.

The website of the National Institute of Diabetes, Digestive, and Kidney Diseases includes a directory of Kidney and Urologic Diseases Organizations; see www.kidney.niddk.nih.gov/resources/organizations.htm. Several of these organizations exist for the sole purpose of supporting patients with specific diseases. Here are some of them.

American Diabetes Association
Attn: National Call Center
1701 North Beauregard Street
Alexandria, VA 22311
Phone: 1-800-DIABETES (1-800-342-2383)
Website: www.diabetes.org

According to their website, the main mission of the American Diabetes Association is "to prevent and cure diabetes and to improve the lives of all people affected by diabetes." The site has extensive information for patients and professionals about diabetes, management of the disease, preventative measures, weight loss, and statistics. The American Diabetes Association also provides grants to help support the salaries of young investigators doing research on diabetes.

American Heart Association
National Center
7272 Greenville Avenue
Dallas, TX 75231
Phone: 1-800-242-8721
Email: Through the website
Website: www.americanheart.org

The website of the American Heart Association provides information on many aspects of cardiovascular disease, including hypertension. One division of the American Heart Association is the American Stroke Association, which provides information on warning signs, prevention, and care for stroke patients.

American Stroke Association
National Center
7272 Greenville Avenue
Dallas, TX 75231
Phone: 1-888-478-7653
Email: Through the website
Website: www.strokeassociation.org

No organization is devoted specifically to glomerulonephritis. The website www.mayoclinic.com provides good information on the disease. In addition, two organizations exist specifically to address two causes of glomerulonephritis: the Alport Syndrome Foundation and IgA Nephropathy Support Network.

Alport Syndrome Foundation
1608 E. Briarwood Terrace
Phoenix, AZ 85048-9414
Phone: 480-460-0621
Website: www.alportsyndrome.org

Alport syndrome is a genetic kidney disease. The mission of the Alport Syndrome Foundation is "to educate and support patients and families that have been affected by Alport Syndrome with the goal of funding research to find more effective treatment protocols and a cure."

IgA Nephropathy Support Network
89 Ashfield Road
Shelburne Falls, MA 01370
Phone: 413-625-9339
Website: www.igansupport.org/index.html

The mission of the IgA Nephropathy Support Network is "to assist patients with IgA nephropathy and their families; to serve as a clearinghouse for dissemination of information about IgA nephropathy; and to promote research for a possible cure." The network provides newsletters and pamphlets.

PKD Foundation
8330 Ward Parkway, Suite 510
Kansas City, MO 64114-2000
Phone: 1-800-PKD-CURE
Email: pkdcure@pkdcure.org
Website: www.pkdcure.org

The best place to obtain useful and reliable information on polycystic kidney disease (PKD) is through the PKD Foundation, which provides educational material for people with PKD, their families, and other interested parties. In addition, it funds grants to researchers who are working to identify the causes of PKD as well as potential treatments and cures for this inherited kidney disease. The PKD Foundation is the only organization in the world that addresses PKD exclusively. I did not discuss ARPKD in this book because most patients have ADPKD. For readers interested in ARPKD, a place to start learning more is found at the link on the PKD Foundation website.

National Kidney Foundation
30 East 33rd St., Suite 1100
New York, NY 10016
Phone: 1-800-622-9010
Email: info@kidney.org
Website: www.kidney.org

The National Kidney Foundation is an organization that provides exceptionally valuable information on kidney diseases in general, as well as on dialysis and transplantation. The NKF offers numerous pamphlets describing many different aspects of kidney failure. This is a useful site for learning basic information about kidney failure.

American Association of Kidney Patients
3505 E. Frontage Rd., Suite 315
Tampa, FL 33607
Phone: 1-800-749-2257
Email: info@aakp.org
Website: www.aakp.org

The American Association of Kidney Patients has a site that is devoted to patient issues. According to their website, the organization "exists to serve the needs, interests, and welfare of all kidney patients and their families. Its mission is to improve the lives of fellow kidney patients and their families by helping them to deal with the physical, emotional, and social impact of kidney disease." The website has extensive information on all aspects of kidney disease.

NUTRITION

As we learned in chapter 5, it can be difficult for a person with kidney disease to eat a proper diet and maintain good nutrition, because of a limited list of permitted foods. This is especially true for anyone on hemodialysis. The American Association of Kidney Patients publishes a useful brochure that lists the sodium, potassium, protein, and caloric content of a wide variety of foods. This brochure can help you in selecting meals that meet the requirements of hemodialysis. You can download it from www.aakp.org/brochures/nutrition-counter.

People on dialysis, especially peritoneal dialysis, generally must have protein supplementation. Liquid supplements designed for dialysis patients are available, but they are expensive. For me, a better alternative was a protein powder derived from egg whites. You can purchase powdered egg whites at www.optimumnutrition.com or at a local GNC. The latter source is often cheaper. Note: *do not buy whey protein.* Derived from dairy products, the product has a high phosphorus content.

The PKD Foundation recently published a cookbook entitled *Brilliant Eats: Simple and Delicious Recipes for Anyone Who Wants to be KidneyWise.* This cookbook is suitable for anyone suffering from chronic kidney disease from any of the major causes. It identifies recipes suitable for people in pre-dialysis, hemodialysis, and peritoneal dialysis, and for people who are considering or preparing for transplant. The book can be purchased at www.kidneywise.org.

TRANSPLANT DONOR WEBSITES

Because there is a shortage of kidneys available for transplantation, efforts are under way to identify more living donors. Several organizations have become increasingly active in matching living donors.

Alliance for Paired Donation
3661 Briarfield Boulevard, Suite 105
Maumee, OH 43537
Phone: 419-866-5505
Email: admin@paireddonation.org
Website: www.paireddonation.org

Through a nationwide computer-matching program, the Alliance for Paired Donation helps arrange for living donations between pairs of potential donors not compatible with the patients with whom they originally intended to donate (see chapter 7). The organization has been in existence for only a few years, but as of this writing, it has arranged seventeen paired donations. Although it does not have agreements with hospitals in all fifty states, it is working to accomplish full coverage. Registering is easy and free.

National Kidney Registry
PO Box 460
Babylon, NY 11702-0460
Phone: 1-800-936-1627
Email: administration@kidneyregistry.org
Website: www.kidneyregistry.org

The National Kidney Registry was founded "to save and improve the lives of people facing kidney failure by increasing the quality, speed, and number of living donor transplants in the world." Although the organization only began its efforts in 2007, it has ambitious plans over the next five years. It wants to provide up to 10,000 living donations per year for those needing a kidney transplant. The cost is free for donors and recipients who work through one of the participating centers. Since February 2008, NKR has facilitated eighty-eight transplants, according to its website.

MatchingDonors.com, Inc.
766 Turnpike Street
Canton, MA 02021
Phone: 781-821-2204
Email: contactus@matchingdonors.com
Website: www.matchingdonors.com

According to its website, the organization was "created to give people in need of transplant surgery an active way to search for a live organ donor. Our goal is to increase the number of transplant surgeries and improve awareness of live organ donation." As the name implies, MatchingDonors.com, Inc., attempts to match prospective living donors with those in need of a transplant. As of January 2010, 1,495 people who are willing to donate kidneys have been listed, and 240 people have registered in need of one. More than 100 transplants have been completed.

Being listed as a patient on the site involves paying a fee. The amount depends on the length of the listing. It ranges from $295 for a monthly membership to $595 for a lifetime membership. Currently, Medicare and insurance companies do not reimburse this expense. For those who cannot afford the fee, Matching Donors claims that it waives it.

If you pursue living donations through any of these websites, you must do so in close consultation with your transplant surgeon. It is not clear from the sites whether those involved in the organization adequately screen potential donors for possible medical conflicts or other disqualifying factors.

FINANCIAL AID

The costs for dialysis and kidney transplantation are substantial. Although some private insurance provides coverage, not all insurance does, and many patients have no private insurance. A major source of funding for dialysis and transplantation comes from the federal government through Medicare and Medicaid. Medicare can provide significant assistance to those in need who meet eligibility requirements. Useful information can be found in the brochure "Medicare Coverage of Kidney Dialysis and Kidney Transplant Services" available at the Medicare website at www.medicare.gov/Publications/Pubs/pdf/10128.pdf. For further information, you can call Medicare at 1-800-MEDICARE (1-800-486-4028). For Medicaid, a joint federal and state program, benefits vary depending on the state and eligibility requirements. Check with your state agency for further information.

The American Kidney Fund provides funds to defray expenses associated with dialysis and transplantation that insurance does not cover. The Fund also provides brochures about kidney function and kidney diseases and educational seminars.

American Kidney Fund
6110 Executive Blvd., Suite 1010
Rockville, MD 20852
Phone: 1-800-638-8299
Email: www.kidneyfund.org/about-us/national-headquarters
Home page: www.kidneyfund.org

Other organizations exist that provide help for transplant costs, including the cost of traveling to the transplant center. A website with a list of some of these organizations and links to them can be found at www.classkids.org/library/resourc/fundraising.htm.

Finally, county services provided by local governments or private organizations also assist in covering such costs of dialysis as transportation, as well as transplantation costs. Check with the social worker at your dialysis or transplant center for guidance.

INDEX

acceptance, 5–6, 66, 160
acidity, 21
acidosis, 21, 60, 63, 163
acyclovir, 139
adrenal glands, 21, 163
advocacy by patients, 10–11, 160
albumin, 104
albuminuria, 33–34, 163
aldosterone, 21, 163
alpha-blockers, 75
Alliance for Paired Donation, 175
Alport Syndrome, 39
Alport Syndrome Foundation, 173
American Association of Kidney
    Patients, 111, 174–75
American Diabetes Association,
    172
American Heart Association, 172
American Kidney Fund, 177
American Stroke Association, 172
Americans with Disabilities Act,
    106
amputations, 31
anemia, 59, 62–63, 104, 163

aneurysms, 46, 163
anger, 5–6
angiotensin I, 20
angiotensin II, 21, 74
angiotensin II receptor antago-
    nists, 74
angiotensin converting enzyme
    (ACE), 74, 163
angiotensin system, 67, 78; and
    regulation of blood pressure,
    20–21, 37–38
angiotensinogen, 20
antibiotics, 80, 137–39
antibodies, 39–40, 76, 133
antifungal agents, 137–39
antigens, 119–20, 164
anti-thymocyte globulin, 138, 146
antiviral agents, 137–39
Aransep, 59
artificial interferon, 151
atenolol, 75
Athena Diagnostics, 46
atherosclerosis, 37, 163
atorvastatin, 139

autosomal dominant polycystic kidney disease (ADPKD), 41–43, 163, 174
autosomal recessive polycystic kidney disease (ARPKD), 41–43, 163, 174

Bactrim, 139
bargaining, 5–6
basilixamab, 138
Baxter International, Inc., 91, 162
beta-blockers, 75
beta cells, 29, 77
Betadyne, 86, 94
bicarbonate, 21
birth defects, 31
blindness, 31
bleeding, 102
blood pressure, regulation of, 21, 35–37, 67
blood typing, 123, 128–29, 164
blood urea nitrogen (BUN), 51, 104, 140–41, 164
biopsy, 57, 164
bone: demineralization, 20, 140; regulating structure of, 22
bone marrow, 22, 164
brain, 33, 75
Bright, Richard, 27

calcidiol, 23, 164
calcitriol, 23, 61, 164
calcium, 50, 164; role in bone health, 22, 104; role in transplant complications, 140; for treating bone loss, 6
calcium acetate, 61

calcium carbonate, 61
calcium-channel blockers, 75
cancer, 72, 78, 139, 152, 155
CAPD. See continuous ambulatory peritoneal dialysis
carbohydrates, 17, 164
carbon dioxide, 17, 164
carbonic acid, 21
cardiovascular disease, 31, 140, 155
catheter, 164; used in hemodialysis, 99–100; used in peritoneal dialysis, 84–87, 94, 109
CCPD. See continuous cyclic peritoneal dialysis
Cellcept, 138
Centers for Disease Control and Prevention, U.S., 31
cholecalciferol, 23, 165
cholesterol, 23, 72–73, 139
chromosomes, 25, 150, 165
clinical trials, 75–79, 141–48
clinicaltrials.gov, 75, 141
clonazepam, 116
clotrimazol troche, 139
clotting, 102
collecting duct, 18
computerized tomography (CT), in diagnosis, 44–45
continuous ambulatory peritoneal dialysis (CAPD), 87–91, 165
continuous cyclic peritoneal dialysis (CCPD), 91–94, 165; traveling and, 106
coping skill(s), 10–15; asking for help, 14–15, 160; believing in recovery, 12, 160; embracing inner strength, 11; feeling in control, 8–9, 160; humor as, 15,

160; moving past denial, 10, 160; and optimism, 13; and priorities, 13, 159–60; and risk-taking, 13–14, 160; and self-advocacy, 10, 160

Cozaar, 74

creatinine, 51–52, 165; and kidney function, 55; levels after transplantation, 140, 147; level versus stability, 57; and peritoneal dialysis, 94

creatinine clearance, 51–52, 95, 165

crossmatch, 133, 165

cyclosporine, 138

cysts, 40–41, 44–46, 78

cytomegalovirus, 139

daclizumub, 138

daily hemodialysis, 97, 162

Darbepoetin, 59

deceased donors, 129–34; blood typing, 132; kidney allocation, 130–33

Deltazone, 138

denial, 5–6, 66, 160

deoxyribonucleic acid (DNA), 25, 165

depression, 5–6

diabetes, 2, 24, 27–34, 49, 67; complications of, 31; and genetic factors, 31–32, 161; prevalence of, 3, 27–28, 30–31; prevention of, 65; role of obesity in, 32–34, 67; and transplant complication, 139, 155; treatment of, 76–77; Type 1, 29–30, 76–77; Type 2, 30–34, 76–77

diabetic nephropathy, 34, 161, 165

dialysate, xii, 84, 91, 94, 165

dialysis, 80–117, 165; basic principles of, 81–83; consent form for, 9; costs of, 177; and diets, 110; and future treatment options, 153–55; and genetic variation, 31–32, 152; and health monitoring, 103–5; history of, 80–81, 83; incidence of, 3–4; prevalence of, 3, 27, 81

dialyzer, 96–97, 154–55, 165

diet, 30, 175; and dialysis, 110–14; to maintain kidney function, 58–59, 67–68

dietitian, 70, 111, 113

diagnosis, 49–64

diastolic blood pressure, 35–37

diuretics, 58, 75

donors: deceased, 129–34; expanded criteria, 132–33; Good Samaritan, 126; living, 124–29; pool of, 125–26; standard criteria, 132–33

drug metabolism, 151

edema, 58, 140, 165

education, 171–74; about kidney disease, 7–9, 66, 159; about treatment options, 50

electrolytes, 16, 166

emotional reactions, 4–7, 9, 10

end-stage renal disease (ESRD), 48, 161; environmental factors in, 26; genetic factors in, 24–26; and Medicare spending, 4; prevalence of, 2; role of obesity in, 67 environmental factors in kidney disease, 26, 30

enzymes, 150–51

Epogen, 59

Epstein-Barr virus, 139, 147

erythrocytes, 16, 22, 104, 166

erythropoietin (EPO), 166; role in erythrocyte production, 22; for treating anemia, 59, 62–63, 104

ESRD. *See* end-stage renal disease

exchange, 166

exercise, 67–68, 140

exit site, 84, 107

expanded criteria donors, 132–33

experimental medications, 75–79

fat, 72–73

fat deposits, 67, 72

fear, 5–6

fenofibrate, 139, 147

financial aid, 177–78

fish oil, 147

fistula, 100–101, 166

fluid retention. *See* edema

free fatty acids, 33

Food and Drug Administration (FDA), 143–44

food labels, 71–73

Fresenius, 162

furosemide, 60

General Nutrition Center (GNC), 106, 175

genes, 24, 78, 166; role in making proteins, 25

gene sequencing, 152–53

Genetic Information Non-discrimination Act of 2008, 47, 153

genetic tests, 46–48; for PKD, 46; and problems associated with insurability, 47

genetics: role in hypertension, 37; role in kidney failure, 24–26; role in PKD, 43–44; role in Type 1 diabetes, 30; role in Type 2 diabetes, 31–32

Gengraf, 138

glomerular diseases, 24, 27, 38–40; incidence of, 3–4; prevalence of, 2; treatment of, 77–78

glomerular filtration rate (GFR), 50, 166; and assessing kidney failure, 52–55, 57, 63; guide for placing dialysis catheters, 98; monitoring transplant function, 141

glomerulus, 18, 38–40, 77, 166

glucose, 28, 50, 76, 84, 95, 166

Good Samaritan donors, 126

Gore-Tex, 100

graft, 100–101, 166

half-life of kidney transplants, 123–24

Healthy Choice, 70, 139

heart disease, 67, 72

hematocrit, 55, 166

hematuria, 50

hemodialysis, 79, 81, 83, 96–105, 166; daily, 97, 153, 162; diets with, 110–15; efficiency of, 102–3; and future treatment

options, 153–55; home, 97; nightly home, 154, 162; and phosphorus restriction, 111, 113; and potassium restriction, 111–13; pros and cons of, 108–17, 153; and sodium restriction, 110–11; and wearable machines, 154, 162
hemoglobin, 50, 55, 166
heparin, 102, 166
hepatitis, 121, 151
herpes, 139
HIV and transplants, 121, 129
HLA typing, 120, 166
home hemodialysis, 97
homeostasis, 17, 166
hormones, 32, 160
Human Genome Project, 25, 150
hydrochlorothiazide, 75
hyperlipidemia, 50, 139, 167
hypertension, 24, 27, 35–38, 48–50, 167; genetic factors in, 37, 161; incidence of, 3–4; prevalence of, 2, 35; prevention of, 65; role of, in other diseases, 67; role of, in transplantation, 140; treatment of, 50, 73–75
Hytrin, 75

immune system: role in glomerular disease, 39–40; role in transplantation, 119–20; role in Type 1 diabetes, 29–30, 76–77
immunoglobulin A (IgA) nephropathy, 39
immunoglobulins, 39
immunosuppressants, 78, 137–40, 142–43, 147, 155

immunosuppression, 77–78, 156–57
incidence of ESRD, 2, 167
infections, 99–100, 106–7, 110, 137–39, 142, 153
inflammation, 33, 38–39, 77
IgA Nephropathy Support Network, 173
inner strength, 11–12
insulin, 28, 29, 76–77, 167; role in glucose metabolism, 28–30
insulin resistance, 32–33, 76, 167
insurance, 128, 154, 177
iron, 104; in restless legs syndrome, 115
islet transplants, 77

Kayexalate, 60
kidney biopsy, 40, 57
kidney disease, stages of, 53–55
kidney donors, 122–34
Kidney Early Evaluation Program, 49–50
kidney failure, 167. See end-stage renal disease (ESRD)
kidney function: evolution of, 17; filtration, 17–20; phosphorous restriction in maintaining, 70; protein restriction in maintaining, 70; salt restriction in maintaining, 69–70
Klonopin, 116
KT/V, 102–3, 167
Kübler-Ross, Elisabeth, 5, 161

Lasix, 60
Lean Cuisine, 70
leptin, 32–33, 167

Lipitor, 139
lisinopril, 74
liver function, 104
living donors, 124–29; evaluation
   of, 127; and Good Samaritan
   donors, 126; and medical costs,
   127–28; number and percentage
   of, 124–25; and surgery, 127.
   See also donors
Loniten, 75
losartan, 74
lupus erythematosus, 39, 77
lymphocytes, 119–20, 167
lymphoma, 139

macroalbuminuria, 33, 163
magnetic resonance imaging
   (MRI), 45, 56
managing kidney failure, 58–61
MatchingDonors.com, 125, 176
Mayo Clinic, 173
Medicaid, 177
medical tourism and transplants,
   126
Medicare, 4, 127–28, 145, 154, 177
Medications: development of,
   150–53; experimental, 75–79
Medrol, 138
metabolism of carbohydrates, 17
metabolites, 16, 167
methylprednisone, 138
microalbuminuria, 34, 163
Microzide, 75
minerals, 73
minoxidil, 75
Mirapex, 116
monounsaturated fats, 72
morphine, 146

mutations, 25–26, 167; in diabetes, 31–32; in PKD, 41–44, 78
Mycelex, 139
mycophenolate mofetil, 138
mycophenolic acid, 138
Myfortic, 138

National Institute of Diabetes,
   Digestive, and Kidney Diseases,
   171
National Institutes of Health, 8,
   30, 35, 66, 80, 141–42, 171
National Kidney Foundation, 49,
   174
National Kidney Registry, 125,
   176
National Library of Medicine, 8,
   171
nausea and vomiting, 62–63
Neoral, 138
nephrologist, 55–58, 70
nephron, 18, 167
nerve damage, 31
New England Program for Kidney
   Exchange, 125
nightly home hemodialysis, 154,
   162
NLM Gateway, 171

obesity, 73, 161; role in diabetes, 4,
   30, 67; role in disease, 26; role
   in hypertension, 38, 67; role in
   kidney failure, 4; and transplants, 121
ondansetron, 62
optimism, 13
Optimum Nutrition, 105, 175
osteoporosis, 22, 140, 155, 167

paired kidney donation, 126–27
pancreas, 30
pancreatic islet cells, 77
panel reactive antibody (PRA), 133, 167
parathyroid hormone, 50, 61, 104, 168
paricalcitol, 61
Patient Protection and Affordable Care Act of 2010, 47, 153
peritoneal dialysis, 81, 83–96, 105–8, 168; efficiency of, 94; exchanges, 87–94; percentage of people using, 105; with polycystic kidney disease, 107; principles of, 83–87; pros and cons of, 105–8, 153; and protein loss, 105; side effects of, 106–7, 153
peritoneal equilibrium test (PET), 95, 168
peritoneal membrane, 83–84
peritonitis, 95–96, 107, 153, 168
pharmacogenetics, 151–52, 168
PhosLo, 61
phosphorus, 17, 50, 60, 73, 104, 168; eliminating, 22; monitoring, 109; and phosphate plaques, 22; restriction of, 70–71, 111; role in bone health, 22; treating high levels of, 60
pirfenidone, 77
pituitary gland, 78
PKD Foundation, 40, 162, 173, 175
polycystic kidney disease (PKD), xi, 2–3, 24, 27, 40–46, 49, 149, 168; diagnosis of, 44–45, 162;

and epithelial cells, 44; and genes, 44; health consequences of, 45–46; incidence of, 3–4; and living donor problems, 126; and mutations, 27, 41–44; prevalence of, 3, 40; peritoneal dialysis in, 107; treatment of, 78–79
polycystin-1, 44
polycystin-2, 44
polygenetic diseases, 31, 168
polyunsaturated fats, 72
potassium, 60, 73, 104, 168; monitoring, 107; restriction, 111
pramipexole, 116
Pravachol, 147
pravastatin, 147
prednisone, 138
prevalence: of diabetes, 27–31; of glomerular diseases, 38; of hypertension, 35; of kidney disease, xi, 2, 168; of polycystic kidney disease, 40
Prinivil, 74
Prograf, 138
proteins, 25, 104, 168; restricting, 70; supplementing, 105, 175
proteinuria, 50
PubMed, 171

Rapamune, 138
Rapamycin, 138
receptors, 32, 168
recovery, 12
Reeve, Christopher, 12
renin, 20, 168
Requip, 116

restless legs syndrome, 114–16, 168
retroviruses, 156
Rocaltrol, 61
ropinirole, 116

scarring, 38–40, 77–78
sensitization in transplantation, 133
signs and symptoms of kidney failure, 61–64
Similect, 138
simvastatin, 139
sirolimus, 78, 138, 147
smoking, 50
social worker, 109
sodium, 72–73, 169; exchange with bicarbonate to balance acidity, 21; and fluid retention, 110–11; restriction, 69–70; role in hypertension, 37–38
sodium bicarbonate, 60
sodium citrate, 60
sodium polystyrene sulfonate, 60
stem cells, 156–57, 162
steroids, 138, 155
strokes, 31, 172
sulfamethoxazole/trimethoprim, 139
systolic blood pressure, 35–37

tacrolimus, 138, 147–48
Tenormin, 75
terazosin, 75
thrombin plasminogen activator, 110
Thymoglobulin, 138, 146
T-lymphocytes, 119, 146, 156

tolvaptan, 78
transplantation, xiii, 78, 118–48, 169; antigen matching, 119–20; candidacy for, 120–22; candidates receiving transplants, 112–23; costs of, 177; crossmatch for, 133; and donors, 122–34; and donor websites, 175–77; in elderly people, 133; and evaluation, 127–29; future approaches to, 155–57; history of, 118–19; and kidney survival, 123–24; and medical tourism, 126; and paired kidney donation, 126–27; and posttransplant care, 137–41; and rejection, 118–20, 133, 137–38, 141–43, 155; and sensitization, 133; surgery, 127, 135–37; and survival, 123–24; waiting for, 134–35, 162
Tricor, 139, 147
triglycerides, 50, 139
tubules, 18
Tums, 61
tunneled, cuffed catheter, 99–100
Type 1 diabetes. See diabetes
Type 2 diabetes. See diabetes

ultrasound, in diagnosis of PKD, 44–45
United Network of Organ Sharing, 122, 124; allocation system for transplants, 130–32, 134
untunneled catheter, 99
urea, 20, 51, 95, 103–4, 169
uremia, 80, 169
ureters, 136, 169

urinalysis, 50, 169
urinary reduction rate (URR), 102–3, 169
urine, production of, 19–20

Valcyte, 139
valganciclovir, 139
vascular accesses for hemodialysis, 98–102; blockage of, 110
vasopressin, 78, 169
vasopressin inhibitor, 78
vitamin D, 17, 22–23, 169; synthesis of, 23; treating low levels of, 61
vitamins, 73; in restless legs syndrome, 115

waiting lists for transplants, 130–32, 135–36
water pills, 75
wearable hemodialysis machines, 154
weight gain, 107, 140
weight loss, 50, 67–68

xenotransplantation, 156, 169

Zemplar, 61
Zenapax, 138
Zestril, 74
Zocor, 139
Zofran, 62
Zovirax, 139

About the Author

Walter A. Hunt, Ph.D., holds a bachelor's degree in chemistry from Bethany College and a doctorate in neuropharmacology from West Virginia University. As a medical researcher for thirty years, he examined the biological basis of diseases never considering that one day he would have to deal with a serious disease of his own. Having polycystic kidney disease (PKD), the fourth leading cause of kidney failure, he suffered seven and a half years of dialysis and two dozen stays in the hospital before receiving the gift of life of a transplant. Now free of kidney problems, Dr. Hunt serves on the Board of Trustees of the PKD Foundation and travels the world.